HONEY
THE NATURE'S GOLD

RECIPES FOR HEALTH

BEES' PRODUCTS SERIES

VOL. I

Mona Illingworth

&

Daniel Andrews

Scarlet Leaf

2017

HONEY – THE NATURE'S GOLD RECIPES FOR HEALTH

SCARLET LEAF PUBLISHING HOUSE

TORONTO ONTARIO CANADA

COPYRIGHT BY Mona Illingworth & Daniel Andrews

ISBN: 978-1-988827-41-4

All rights reserved.

No part of this book can be used or reproduced in any manner whatsoever without written permission, except in the case of brief quotations embodied in critical articles and reviews.

For information address:

Scarlet Leaf Publishing House:

scarletleafpublishinghouse@gmail.com

HONEY – THE NATURE'S GOLD RECIPES FOR HEALTH

We dedicate this book to our parents, for their love and support

HONEY – THE NATURE'S GOLD RECIPES FOR HEALTH

HONEY – THE NATURE'S GOLD RECIPES FOR HEALTH

Table of Contents

Introduction 17
Part 1 - About Bees and Honey 22
   Chapter 1 22
   A Short History of Honey 22
   Chapter 2 29
   About Bees 29
   Chapter 3 35
   About Honey 35
      Physical Properties 36
      Biochemical composition 39
      Classification of Honey 45
         Ordering by floral source 45
         Systematization by processing and packaging 46
      How to buy quality honey 48
      Honey's Healing Features 50
Part 2 - Honey Therapy 59
   Chapter 4 59
   Respiratory diseases 59
      Asthma 59
         Recipe 1 - Honey and Water 61
         Recipe 2 - Honey and Milk 63
         Recipe 3 - Honey and Lemon 65

Recipe 4 - Honey and Grapefruit Juice...................67

Recipe 5 - Honey and Cinnamon..............................69

Bronchitis 71

Recipe 6 - Honey and Turmeric..............................73

Recipe 7 - Honey, Lemon and Black Radish 75

Recipe 8 - Honey and Apple Cider Vinegar 78

Recipe 9 - Honey and Thyme 80

Recipe 10 - Honey and Cloves.................................82

Acute Pharyngitis 84

Common Cold (Nasopharyngitis) 84

Recipe 11 - Honey and Sunflower Seed Powder....86

Recipe 12 - Honey, Fenugreek and Ginger.............88

Recipe 13 - Honey, Ginger and Black Pepper.........91

Recipe 14 - Honey, Lemon and Ginger...................94

Acute Tonsillitis (Sore Throat)..97

Recipe 15 - Honey, Lemon and Red Onion 98

Recipe 16 - Honey and Indian Gooseberries (Alma) 101

Recipe 17 - Honey, Garlic and Olive Oil 103

Recipe 18 - Honey and Safflower..........................106

Recipe 19 - Honey, Bitter Gourd and Great Basil. 108

Chapter 5...110

Cardio-vascular Diseases...110

Arterial Hypertension (High Blood Pressure)...........110

Recipe 20 - Honey and Cucumber........................112

Recipe 21 - Honey and Dill Seeds 114

Recipe 22 - Honey and Caraway 116

Recipe 23 - Honey and Great Basil 118

Recipe 24 - Honey and Garlic 120

Recipe 25 - Honey, Walnuts and Elderberry Flowers 122

Recipe 26 - Honey, Red Beets, Lemon and Carrot 125

Coronary Artery Disease (Ischemic Heart Disease) .. 128

Recipe 27 - Honey, Corn Oil and Egg White 130

Recipe 28 - Honey and Horseradish 132

Recipe 29 - Honey and Common Sea Buckthorn . 134

Recipe 30 - Honey, Lemon, Red Onion and Garlic 136

Recipe 31 - Honey, Lemon and Garlic 139

Cardiac Insufficiency (Heart Failure) 142

Recipe 32 - Honey and Cheese 144

Recipe 33 - Honey and Oats 145

Cardiomyopathy 147

Recipe 34 - Honey and Common St John's Wort . 149

Varicose veins (varicosities) 151

Recipe 35 - Honey and Garlic 152

Recipe 36 - Honey and Apple Cider Vinegar 154

Recipe 37 - Honey and Red Onion Juice 156

Peripheral artery disease 158

Recipe 38 - Honey and European Mistletoe 160

Recipe 39 - Honey and Dog Rose 162

Recipe 40 - Honey and Fresh Beer Yeast 164

Recipe 41 - Honey and Dried Beer Yeast 166

Chapter 6 168

Digestive Diseases 168

Mouth Ulcers 168

Gingivitis 169

Recipe 42 - Honey and Cinnamon 170

Recipe 43 - Honey and Liquorice 172

Gastro-Esophageal Reflux Disease (GERD) 175

Recipe 44 - Honey and Chamomile 177

Gastritis 179

Recipe 45 - Honey and Cinnamon 181

Peptic Ulcer Disease (Gastric and Duodenal Ulcer) 183

Recipe 46 - Honey and Ginger 185

Recipe 47 - Honey, Liquorice and Chamomile 187

Dyspepsia (Indigestion) 190

Recipe 48 - Honey and Apple Cider Vinegar 192

Biliary Lithiasis (Gallstones) 194

Recipe 49 - Honey and Liquorice 196

Recipe 50 - Honey and Dog Rose 198

Recipe 51 - Honey and Watermelon Rind 200

Constipation 202

Recipe 52 - Honey and Liquorice 204

Recipe 53 - Honey, Walnuts and Aloe 206

Obesity 209
    Recipe 54 - Honey, Lemon and Cinnamon 211
    Recipe 55 - Honey and Beer Yeast 214
    Recipe 56 - Honey and Dill Seeds 216

Chapter 7 218

Kidney Diseases 218

  Urinary Tract Infections.. 218
    Recipe 57 - Honey, Garlic and Apple Cider Vinegar 220
    Recipe 58 - Honey, Lemon, Olive Oil, and Parsley Root 223
    Recipe 59 - Honey, Lemon and Carrot Juice 226
    Recipe 60 - Honey, Apple and Dog Rose Juice 228
    Recipe 61 - Honey and Celery Seeds 230
    Recipe 62 - Honey and Dog Rose Seeds 232

  Renal Lithiasis (Kidney Stones) 234
    Recipe 63 - Honey, Elderberry Flowers, and Lemon 236
    Recipe 64 - Honey, Cucumber, Carrot, Black Radish and Red Beets 239
    Recipe 65 - Honey and Corn Silk (macerate) 243
    Recipe 66 - Honey and Corn Silk (infusion) 245
    Recipe 67 - Honey and Corn Silk (decoction) 247
    Recipe 68 - Honey and Green Walnuts 249

  Benign Prostatic Hyperplasia (Prostate Gland Enlargement) 251

Recipe 69 - Honey and Pumpkin Seeds 253

Recipe 70 - Honey, Horseradish and Lemon 255

Recipe 71 - Honey and Celery Juice 258

Recipe 72 - Honey, Carrots, Walnuts and Turmeric 260

Chapter 8 263

Endocrine Diseases 263

Menopause 263

Recipe 73 - Honey and Liquorice (infusion) 264

Recipe 74 - Honey and Hawthorn (infusion) 266

Amenorrhea 268

Recipe 75 - Honey and Common Yarrow 270

Recipe 76 - Honey and Caraway 272

Dysmenorrhea (Menstrual cramps) 274

Recipe 77 - Honey and Corn Silk 276

Recipe 78 - Honey and Dill 278

Hypocalcaemia 280

Recipe 79 - Honey and Chicken Egg Shells 282

Recipe 80 - Honey, Chicken Egg Shells and White Wine 284

Osteoporosis 286

Recipe 81 - Honey, Garlic and Apple Cider Vinegar 288

Recipe 82 - Honey, Chicken Egg Shells and Lemon 291

Chapter 9 294
Nervous System Diseases 294

Anxiety 294
Recipe 83 - Honey and Hawthorn (macerate) 296
Recipe 84 - Honey and Celery Juice 298

Anorexia 300
Recipe 85 - Honey, Red Wine and Horseradish ... 302
Recipe 86 - Honey and Dates 304

Alzheimer's Disease 306
Recipe 87 - Honey and European Blueberry 308
Recipe 88 - Honey, Onion Juice and Black Pepper 310
Recipe 89 - Honey and Orange Juice 313

Depression 315
Recipe 90 - Honey and Common Sea Buckthorn . 317
Recipe 91 - Honey and Onion 319

Chronic Fatigue Syndrome 321
Recipe 92 - Honey, Green Walnuts and Dog Rose 323
Recipe 93 - Honey, Green Walnuts and Cloves 326
Recipe 94 - Honey, Carrots and Celery Juice 329
Recipe 95 - Honey and Liquorice (decoction) 332

Chapter 10 334
Skin Diseases 334

Acne 334
Recipe 96 - Honey and Liquorice Powder 336

Recipe 97 - Honey and Potato 339

Recipe 98 - Honey and Apple 341

Recipe 99 - Honey, Yoghurt and Lemon 343

Eczema (Atopic Dermatitis) 345

Recipe 100 - Honey and Cinnamon 347

Recipe 101 - Honey and Cucumber 349

Recipe 102 - Honey, Aloe and Liquorice Powder . 351

Psoriasis 354

Recipe 103 - Honey and Dried/Fresh Beer Yeast . 356

Recipe 104 - Honey and Turmeric 358

Skin Infections 360

Recipe 105 - Honey and Yoghurt for Genital Yeast Infection in Women 360

Chapter 11 362

Arthritis 362

Recipe 106 - Honey and Cinnamon 364

Recipe 107 - Honey and Caraway 366

Recipe 108 - Honey, Ginger, Garlic and Apple Cider Vinegar 368

Recipe 109 - Honey and Corn Silk (infusion) 371

Recipe 110 - Honey, Green Walnuts and Ginger . 373

Recipe 111 - Honey and Liquorice (macerate) 376

Chapter 12 379

Anemia 379

Recipe 112 - Honey, Aloe and Red Wine 381

Recipe 113 - Honey and Milk 383

Recipe 114 - Honey and Green Walnuts 385

Recipe 115 - Honey, Walnuts and Lemon 387

Recipe 116 - Honey and Red Beets 390

Chapter 13 392

Eye Diseases 392

Conjunctivitis (Pink Eye) 392

Recipe 117 - Honey and Water 394

Visual Acuity 396

Recipe 118 - Honey, Carrot and Lemon 397

Recipe 119 - Honey and Liquorice 400

Recipe 120 - Honey, Walnuts and Lemons 403

Cataract 406

Recipe 121 - Honey and Water 408

Recipe 122 - Honey and Breckland Wild Thyme (Creeping Thyme) for early stages of Cataracts ... 410

Chapter 14 412

Conclusion 412

Bibliography 415

Authors' Bio 427

Introduction

Little I knew as a child, when lying on the green, fat grass on the field, watching the flying of the bees from flower to flower and hearing their monotonous, yet soothing buzz, that one day I'll end up writing a book on these tiny creatures and honey, their marvelous product.

Although born and brought up in a big city, as a child, I used to spend most of my holidays in the country, at my grandparents'. They lived at the foothills of some wild, enchanting mountains, so I had the privilege to see firsthand how the relation between humans and nature transforms itself in the products necessary for the daily living. And, at the same time, I learned to watch this connection with reverence and to participate into it with joy, while carrying on with readying the ground for sowing, planting the seeds, harvesting the crops and the hay, tending to the animals, as well as accomplishing the various housework, such as traditional bread making in a classical brick oven - I can still smell the wonderful fragrance of the bread fresh out of the oven - and transforming the fruits and vegetables into delicious and nurturing marmalades, jams, syrups, various preserves and pickles.

Now, granny was a wise woman with a genuine grasp and well-rounded familiarity in terms of the use of honey, medicinal plants, and other natural products. Her enthusiasm and adroitness in such topics, as well as her knowledge, have found their way to me, marveled me and stuck with me over the years.

Later on, when I met Daniel, and, in the beginning, accidentally engaged in discussing natural products features, I was surprised and delighted to discover a kindred spirit. After a while, following many conversations during which we both deplored the too little employment of all these wonderful and beneficial natural goods, an idea slowly took form in our minds. All this knowledge from which humans took so much advantage over the centuries, but unfortunately largely slipped away from ongoing use, should be handed over to people again, so that they can learn these things and start once more to apply them.

Moreover, the fact that we are both medical doctors, actually helped in creating a bridge between traditional medicine and the natural way.

Thus, this project, which includes a series of books, emerged. The books to follow will deal with the other bee products from the point of view of therapy, cosmetics, household and kitchen use.

How should this book be read? In our opinion, we feel the reading of the book should proceed in the order it was conceived, to achieve a better understanding and to gain the maximum benefit. Furthermore, in the next lines we will briefly describe the various sections of the book.

Since the very beginning of the book, we decided on writing a short honey history because, on one hand, we noticed that many people are pretty unaware of the long and beneficial use of this marvel, and, on the other hand, we believe it is a quite fascinating, worth-to-be-developed theme. We hope the facts will appeal to you too.

Next, we dedicated a chapter to the bees themselves. We feel this would be the least one can do to honor these little creatures who offered mankind so many valuable gifts over the time.

Moreover, we believe the amazing data concerning their lives pays the effort to read this chapter.

In the next section, we deal with honey's characteristics on the whole: physical and chemical properties, classifications and advice regarding honey purchase. We allotted an entire chapter to therapeutic features, and basic traits, mechanisms, and corresponding diseases.

For the recipes chapters, we agreed on adding short depictions of diseases, specifically a short definition followed by symptoms, with and without signs, and, in the end, the risk factors. We found this step helpful, in order to offer a better understanding of the conditions to be treated. The corresponding recipes follow after each illness.

In composing the recipes, we employed mostly those already known and used in our families and by friends and acquaintances, but we also selected and adjusted recipes from other trustworthy sources. In this pursuit, we carefully weighed the ingredients, specified their amounts, the preparation methods and, if required, the overall duration of the cure and the eventual repetition. We checked up and wrote down the components, their features, and their effects on various diseases for each ingredient.

We also considered the necessity of adding the possible adverse effects of the ingredients, the associated conditions in which they are contraindicated, and also the already known interactions with the medical drugs. To fulfill this task, we deployed an extensive research regarding all these topics.

We favored a friendly voiced language, therefore the information conveyed is as accessible as possible to anybody, regardless of their educational level.

At the very end of the book, beyond the recipes part, you will find a condensed conclusion and a bibliography section.

Yet again, we stress the fact that we wrote this book to raise awareness about honey and other natural plants, and about their preparation. As such, this book is a guide, and we highlight the importance of observing the indicated amounts of ingredients and the notes regarding their adverse effects and contraindications, particularly by people suffering from multiple diseases.

We advise the complete exclusion of other sugars from the diet, while following a treatment with honey. We mention that we take no responsibility for the way the recipes are used or for any adverse effects. We also advocate seeking medical advice before starting any treatment described in the book and medical supervision during the treatment.

Last, but not least, we thank you for purchasing this book. Enjoy!

Mona Illingworth and Daniel Andrews

Part 1 - About Bees and Honey

Chapter 1

A Short History of Honey

When we think about honey, a particular image often comes to mind. It is a picture about a fine, intricate network, connecting humans with bees and flowers over the millennia. This web stretches itself a long way back in time, towards the beginning of flowering plants and insects on Earth. We invite you in a fascinating voyage over the folds of this canvas.

Once upon a time, the very first bees appeared and they actually looked more like wasps. Anyway, solitary bees were first encountered in the fossil remains from Eocene, around 56-34 million years ago. Some of the oldest documented species of bee date from Upper Oligocene (towards 23 million years ago): Apis aquitaniensis was discovered in Aix en Provence (France), Apis (Synapis) cuenoti in Cereste, Vaucluse, France, and in Rott, Germany, were found the species Apis dormitans and Apis (Synapis) henshawi. Other populations of fossil bees, such as Synapis petrefacta bee from Bohemia, cover the periods from Oligocene to Miocene in the western world. Only much later, in Miocene (23-5 million years ago), appear the first honey-gathering social bees.

Thus, a close, vital connection emerged. The flowers depended on the bees for pollination, and vice versa, the bees needed the flowers for their golden crop. Consequentely, a perfect fabric appeared and man got himself interwoven in this fabric.

Probably, early humans realized many of honey's benefits soon. Hence, the gold rush began.

Initially, men spotted and robbed the wild bee nests. At first, they defended themselves with water, and, later, they used smoke. Depictions of such activities can still be seen in cave paintings such as those found in Spain and dating as far as 7000 B.C. Anyway, this hunting occupation stretches over centuries and is still practiced in certain regions of Asia and Africa.

Undoubtedly, bee lifestyle and behaviour were thoroughly and precisely studied over the time. And lastly, our great-grandfathers came up with ingenious methods to bring the bees close to their homes. In the beginning, they cut the tree truncheons containing bee nests and put them near their homes. Later on, they constructed hives from various materials, such as twigs woven into baskets or river stone pipes, all held together by clay. An illustration of such a primitive beekeeping is represented by the 30-intact hives dating around 900 B.C., discovered by the archaeologist Amihai

Mazar of Jerusalem's Hebrew University in the ruins of the city of Rehov (North of Israel).

Proofs of honey consumption have been found all over the antique world. Wild honey, along with meat and, of course, fruits were most probably among the first foods used by people. For instance, in Rig Veda, one of most sacred book in India dating around 3000 BC, honey is mentioned many times in various drugs, as well as an ingredient in different festivities.

In the 2nd millennia people already knew 8 types of honey with particular features, so that each was recommended in certain illnesses. Also, honey's use was finely entangled with religious life, its knowledge (Madhu vidya) being attributed to Asvins, the twin gods of medicine and healing. Vishnu and Krishna are often called in texts Madhava (the nectar-born ones), word derived from that of *bee*, probably due to its love for order and diligence.

In addition, in another great oriental civilization, namely the Assiro-Babylonian, honey found its place in various realms, especially in medicine. Almost 5000-year-old clay tablets mention the use of honey as medicine, and archaeological works uncovered clay pots on which ancient hands wrote honey-based ointment recipes. And of course, one should not forget the stipulations regarding honey's utility as a therapy. These specifications were well depicted in Hammurabi's Code (the Babylonian Code). All these mentions highlight the huge importance of this ingredient in the Mesopotamian culture.

Furthermore, Talmud, the large collection of writings of rabbinic Judaism, contains lots of referrals to the healing benefits of honey, in combination with water, milk or even with wine mixtures. And, let's not forget that Mosses's promised land was precisely one of "*milk and honey*".

Jumping back again towards west, one encounters the first proof of an apiary in the Sun temple near Cairo, a construction dating from 2400 B.C. As a matter of fact, bee was held in great esteem all over the ancient Egypt. The pharaohs honored it, and, moreover, it was often seen as a symbol of royalty. Depictions of bees can also be found in the hieroglyphs and they prove such veneration.

The ancient Egyptians used honey in many ways, in the kitchen as a sweetener for cookies, as a particular form of yeast for bread, and as a special ingredient in alcoholic beverages. They not only knew how to use honey to preserve fruits, but also how to obtain honey-based beautifying products.

Besides, honey cakes were considered as adequate offerings to the gods. The pharaoh Ramses III laid 15 tons of honey at the feet of Hapi, the god of the Nile, as an atonement.

Honey represented an important embalming ingredient and a suitable gift for the dead, as shown by the vessels with honey from pharaoh Tutankhamen's tomb. It is amazing that, despite being over 3000 years old, the honey was still edible at the time of discovery.

And that's not all. Honey was mentioned in the 5000-year-old Imhotep's medical treatise, as well. The famous Imhotep, to whom the old Egyptians finally granted a divine status, is considered by many historians to be the real father of medicine. In his treatise, he minutely describes treatments and recipes with honey. All of them were passed down for countless generations.

Later on, in Historia Animalium, Aristotle recommends beeswax and propolis in wound treatment. Subsequently, Hippocrates, the well-known physician of ancient Greece, appraises honey and its product propolis as the dearest medicines. In his works, he recognizes the anti-inflammatory features of honey and highlights its role in preventive medicine.

Similarly, the antique Greeks considered honey a valuable and important aliment. There were many honey cookies and sweets, such as kykeon, a dish containing honey mixed with cheese and barley flour. However, honey was a luxury product and was served only on banquets.

Because of its importance, honey found its place in the Greek mythology, as well. It was said that the bees from Mount Ida had created a special honey just to feed Zeus. They also cooked special crescent-formed cookies as offerings for the goddess Artemis.

Finally, there were many traditions associated with honey. In order to ensure harmony between spouses and good relationship with the mother in law, the bride was supposed to dip her fingers in honey and smear the house's threshold with it.

Likewise, Romans used honey as offering for gods, in medicine and, obviously, in cooking. Romans also knew the art of food preservation with honey. Hence, "*Honey's apples*" was the poetic name for quinces held in honey.

During the Roman Empire, beekeeping literally flourished. Pliny the Elder extensively describes in his works the various employments of honey and other bees' products in cosmetics, medicine, and household items, such as writing tablets or candles.

In fact, from 900 medical remedies known to Roman medicine, about 500 involved the use of honey. Honey, along with milk, were offered at tombs on February 21st (the day of the dead), and Romans gifted one another white vessels with honey on the first day of the year.

Actually, in ancient Rome honey was so much valued that it was even considered as means of exchange instead of gold. This tradition continued later, over the centuries, until the Middle Ages.

Subsequently, honey further held a great importance well after the Dark Ages. In Europe, it was part of diet in various forms, such as cookies, honeycombs, and beverages, both alcoholic (mead) and non-alcoholic (milk or tea with honey).

It is worth noticing the importance given to nectar during these times. It became as precious as salt, and for centuries remained a notable commercial item.

Toward the end of Middle Ages, apiaries were founded in almost all the monasteries. Along with the various use of honey in so many fields, Christianity led to a higher production of beeswax, due to the ever-increasing amount necessary for candle making.

On other continents, people used it in various foods, rituals and medicines, too. Numerous proofs from the Australian continent point to the fact that the Aborigines have used honey for a long time.

Far away, on the American continent, the Mayans used a ritual beverage from Lonchocarpus tree bark and honey. Nowadays, the indigenes from the Amazon basin, as well as from different African countries, still have knowledge in the various use of honey.

Unfortunately, with the cultivation of sugar cane in large plantations beginning with the 18th century, and later on with the ever-increasing development of pharmaceuticals, a gradual and significant decline in honey use as a sweetener in foods and beverages occurred. A similar decline was noted in medicine.

Nevertheless, since the end of the past century, the development of health oriented movements has brought in the foreground the multiple benefits of honey once more. In this way, nature's gold has regained gently but perceptibly its important and well deserved place in various spheres of human's life.

Chapter 2

About Bees

We feel that a special chapter should be dedicated to these amazing insects, the bees. On one hand, they present remarkable features, worthy of being known. On the other hand, over time, human beings benefited enormously from their gold in so many areas.

So, let's verify together who actually are these tiny and beautiful creatures. We promise not to become (too) boring.

For start, there are about 20,000 species of bees, from which honey producing species, including stingless honey bees, represent only a very small number. However, true honey bees belong to genus *Apis*, with seven existent species at the time being. Nowadays, *Apis mellifera* lives on many continents, in Europe, in Africa and in the Middle East.

Honey bees prosper in large, well-structured communities/colonies, feature which classify them as social insects. What does that actually mean? That indicates that they display particular behaviours, which contribute to their successful way of life and a few of them are: labor division, communication, defense, and elaborate nest construction. Some voices affirm that due to such characteristics, bee communities should be considered a super-organism. Furthermore, many resemble their organization to a caste system too. Now, isn't that captivating?

Let's take a closer look to a typical honey bee colony. One queen or the sexually mature female reigns over the entire community, except during swarming periods, when there may coexist more than one queen in a particular bee colony. The majority of community is represented by more than 50,000 workers or sexually immature females. A third type of member is the drone, the sexually developed male, ranging from a few to several hundred, depending on the population and time of the year.

To begin with, the queen looks different from the other members of the colony, with a longer body, shorter wings, and longer and curved stinger. Her lifespan is normally 2 to 3 years, and her main function consists in laying eggs in order to ensure the next generations. We're talking about an impressive number of eggs, up to a quarter of a million eggs in a year.

She also fulfils another major role through pheromone production, substances which act as a social unifier and thus individualize a colony. Their distribution, as well as the communicative "bee dances", control the survival connected activities. Back to the queen, she is constantly fed and pampered by the worker bees, and that's really a crucial issue, because good and enough food, as well as the number of beeswax cells, determine the number of laid eggs.

Finally, one more thing about queens. As already mentioned, at times, an old queen coexists for a while with new queens. The latter originate from less than 3 days old worker larvae or from fertilized eggs in one of the following situations: in emergency, when the queen gets lost or killed; while swarming, to ensure the creation of new colonies; or in case of supersedure, to replace an aging and failing queen.

In turn, the most numerous members of the community, the workers, are the smallest bees. They are provided with specialized, particular glands such as scent glands, brood food glands, and abdominal wax glands, as well as with pollen baskets. All these structures are essential in carrying on the hive's labors.

The young adults are involved in lots of works: nest building - beeswax combs and brood rearing, hive cleaning and ventilating, handling the newly brought nectar and guarding.

In opposition, the more mature field bees participate in foraging for pollen, propolis, and nectar. During summer, these bees live 6 weeks on average. Nevertheless, the autumn generations of workers may live up to 6 months, so that the colony overcomes winter and secures a new generation in spring.

Additionally, the male bees, or the drones, are the largest members of the community, with the largest head but with no stinger, no wax glands or pollen baskets. In general, there are up to 500 drones in a hive and they are born only in summer. Their major role is performed during the mating flight, when they fertilize the new queens. It seems they do no other work in the hive, nor do they gather food from flowers. However, many consider their presence to be essential for the normal function of the colony.

Towards winter, when the cold settles, the accent falls on food preservation in the hive. And as drones eat 3 times the amount of food the workers need, they are driven out from the hive and find their end in the cold weather of that time of the year.

Lastly, the bees' brood starts with the eggs, which are laid by the queen, one in each cell. After two days, they hatch and the larvae appear. The adult worker bees feed them for about 6 days, when they turn into pupae. In this stage, the brood gradually gains adult forms. At the end of around 13 days, new workers, drones and queens come out.

The bee food consists in a combination of pollen and nectar. In fact, pollen represents the only source of protein and fat for bees. One adult worker bee requires about 4 mg of pollen daily. Some pollen constituents, in particular amino acids and vitamins, are essential to rear brood, or to significantly increase its number. Just for the record, a few such amino acids are valine, lysine, leucine, and isoleucine, and important vitamins are represented by B vitamins, especially pyridoxine, which is pretty abundant in royal jelly, as well as the fat-soluble vitamins A, D, E, and K. Last but not least, phytosterol represents a very important fat in the bees' diet.

Furthermore, nectar embodies the main source of sugars and water in bees' nutrition. Its sugar composition includes sucrose, fructose and glucose.

An adult worker requires on average about 4 mg sugar per day. It is important to note that there is a high amount of water in nectar, and this is required and enough for the many processes in the hive's economy (internal balance, food preparation and hive maintenance). Only during very hot summer days the worker bees have to bring extra water from puddles or small lakes.

Finally, bees carry on complex, season-dependent activities. The most interesting is swarming. This phenomenon occurs especially in spring, and leads to the creation of new colonies, usually just one, but occasionally more than one.

A swarm numbers from thousands to tens of thousands of bees. In wilderness, a new colony is founded at tens of meters from the original one for a few days. Then, scout bees are sent to explore the surroundings. When they return, they bring a new location for the nest of the new bees' community.

In the end, it is of huge interest to highlight an important activity, pollination, which bees carry on year after year. This endeavour ensures the survival of countless plant species, except for a few ones, such as corn, wheat and rice, which rely on the wind or self-pollination.

We need to point out that a significant decline in honey bee populations would jeopardize food availability for humankind. That brings to the forefront the importance of the relatively newly described colony collapse disorder (CCD), characterized precisely by a slow decline in the bee stocks in the western countries over the years.

Research upon the causes of this condition revealed it as being rather a syndrome, not a disease, consequence of combined effects of many factors. The gathered data suggest first of all the involvement of neonicotinoids, a class of pesticides introduced about 20 years ago, against crop pests, which paralyze the nervous system and cause the death of the insects, including the bees. Then, possible culprits are viruses such as Israeli acute paralysis virus, tobacco ring spot virus and the deformed wing virus, as well as parasites, among them *Apocephalus borealis* and the *varroa mite*.

Up to date, there have been no proposals for effective prophylactic measures against CCD. However, an ever-increasing number of better informed people means a higher chance in finding solutions for this threatening situation. And that is the very reason why we found it more than appropriate to include this information here.

Chapter 3

About Honey

The first chapter of honey creation begins with the tireless bees flying over the fields and forests and gathering the flowers' nectar, pollen and propolis. And in order to accomplish this mission, bees cover about 48,000 miles for just 1 liter of honey, as pointed by a beekeeper in 1911.

In bees' nests, the nectar undergoes a complex processing, involving the worker bees, which are also responsible for other important hive-related tasks. Finally, the quality of the emerging honey is based on acquired physical features, as well as on chemical composition, which, in turn, depend largely on many factors, such as the type of flora from which the nectar comes, the bee colony strength, the various environmental conditions, the climate and, of course, the human honey processing.

Physical Properties

Let's first concisely verify honey's physical features and, here comes the important part, their practical applications.

To begin with, honey thickness or viscosity relies on its water content and also on its temperature. Now, water load in honey is pretty low. It represents less than 20%, compared to the sugar amount, which makes up about 70%.

There are over 20 sugars in honey, and fructose represents more than half of the total amount, whereas glucose comprises less than half. Due to this high sugar load, at room temperature, glucose undergoes granulation and crystallization, and, consequently, the glucose crystals float in other sugars and components. In this form, the melting point is only around 40°C, and honey appears like a viscous liquid.

The practical importance of this property occurs in honey harvesting, where the thicker the honey is, the more challenging the extraction becomes.

Furthermore, honey is quite hygroscopic, which means it absorbs water from the air. This trait is particularly important for honey storage, as a higher water content enables the yeast, a natural component of honey, to start fermentation. That's why honey may be pasteurized at 70°C. At this temperature, this yeast is killed. However, when pasteurization is unwanted or not possible, honey should be kept in tightly sealed containers, thus avoiding the infiltration of water vapors from the atmosphere in the honey.

Depending on the water load, there are shifts in the values of the honey refractive index, measured with a refractometer. Commonly, this index starts from a value of 1.5, corresponding to a water content of 13%, and can reach 1.47, namely 25% water load.

Next, honey exerts an effect on the polarized light, or otherwise said, it exhibits optical properties, because of its content in sugars. This characteristic is measured by means of the mixture ratio or the overall rotation of the polarization plane, ratio which results mainly from the fructose and glucose effects, the former causing a negative rotation, and the latter inducing a positive one.

In addition, honey composition includes different amounts of acids and minerals, in other words electrolytes, so that it displays various degrees of electrical conductivity.

Practically, the two water-related honey features, the effect on the polarized light and also its electrical conductivity, measured as ash content, are all characteristics employed to establish the quality of honey.

Finally, honey shows particular thermal characteristics because of its sugar load. Heating leads to caramelization of honey, and, depending on the overall composition, this process begins at 70°C, and reaches 110°C. Acids content lowers even further this temperature.

The darkening of honey occurs over a few months at a slow pace at room temperature or very quickly through heating. This phenomenon is also due to the amino acids included in honey, and can be delayed by cold storage.

It is extremely important to keep in mind that heating can greatly affect the composition and properties of honey, including aroma, flavor, color, etc. and cause alteration and denaturation of various components, such as pollen, propolis, enzymes, anti-oxidants, vitamins, and amino acids. That's why heating should be altogether avoided or at least carried out for very short amounts of time and at the lowest possible temperatures. This is also the very reason why, in all recipes, we advise adding the honey after the cooling of the mixture and avoiding its thermal preparation.

Biochemical composition

Still, let's take a closer look at the biochemical make-up of this golden treasure. In fact, this complex combination includes over 180 different types of substances, including sugars, proteins, minerals, vitamins, antioxidants, enzymes, antimicrobial factors, propolis, nectar etc. As already mentioned in the beginning of the chapter, there are many variations in its structure, depending on numerous factors.

Essentially, honey is a sugar suspension, in which simple sugars, monosaccharides fructose and glucose have the highest percentages, about 38% and respectively, around 31%, while more complex sugars, specifically oligosaccharides (maltose, sucrose) and other carbohydrates, are present in low amounts (in total 10 %). However, it is precisely this reduced quantity of complex sugars that are mainly responsible for the existence of different honey types, as they determine the color, flavor and taste.

The proportion of these sugars depends on the geographical regions, too. It should also be noted that, compared to blossom honey, honeydew honey incorporates larger amounts of complex sugars. The exact proportion of each sugar can be determined using different methods of chromatography.

If we compare honey to the refined table sugar, both from sugar cane and sugar beets, only raw, natural honey preserves all its components, such as proteins, enzymes, vitamins, etc. Subsequently, it retains its entire healing and therapeutic qualities. Cane and beet-sugars, due to processing, are deprived of these qualities. Consequently, these refined sugars bring only "empty calories" to the human body.

There is also another factor worth mentioning here, the glycemic index. It is a parameter whose values show the impact of ingested sugar on the level of the blood sugar. For honey, the glycemic index has a wide variation, from 32 to 85, while for sugar it lies around 65.

The organic acids (about 1%), the major one being the gluconic acid, along with smaller quantities of formic, acetic, lactic, succinic, malic, maleic, pyroglutamic, citric acid, etc. are other important elements found in honey.

Bees supplement most acids. Therefore, nearly all honeys are acidic, with a pH value under 7, generally varying between 3.4 and 4.6. It reaches a particular value of up to 6 in chestnut honey, but with still higher values in honeydew honeys (over 6).

Regarding density, honey is about 35 % heavier than water, with the density measuring approximately 1.36 kg/l.

Similarly, amino acids and proteins make up a small amount, of about 0.5%. Nevertheless, all physiologically essential amino acids are included. Besides, the amino acid proline helps in assessing honey's ripeness. Its value normally exceeds 200 mg/kg, and values under 180 mg/kg arise suspicions of adulteration with sugar. Enzymes make up most of the proteins in honey: diastase (amylase), which turns starch into maltose; invertase, involved in the conversion of sucrose into fructose and glucose; catalase and glucose oxidase, which adjust the synthesis of an anti-bacterial factor, etc.

Diastase and invertase are also good parameters in assessing honey quality and particularly its freshness, as their activity decreases with storage and heating. Yet, the best parameter for quality evaluation is HMF (Hydroxy-methyl-furfuraldehyde), a product resulting from fructose decay. It accumulates with prolonged heat and storage.

Standards have been developed for the HMF values. In conformity with International Food Standard and European norms, the maximum is normally of 40 mg/kg, whereas honey from tropics should have an HMF of up to 80 mg/kg.

Vitamins and minerals form a pretty tiny amount of up to 0.3 % in honey's composition. There are only some traces of vitamins C and B complex. Regarding minerals, potassium represents about a third of all minerals, along with a large spectrum of other minerals and trace elements, calcium, magnesium, iron, copper, chromium, selenium, manganese, molybdenum, sulphur, iodine, etc.

Usually, depending especially on the botanical source of honey, darker honey is richer in trace elements. Nonetheless, sometimes light types of honey may show a higher content.

As already mentioned, the honey type, color and taste depend on the botanical source and on composition, chiefly on sugars, but also on amino acids and acids. Honey aroma, instead, is determined by volatile substances, most of them from the plant, and some produced by the bees. These volatile substances number up to around 600 in various honeys.

Other compounds, the polyphenols, include many biochemical component types, primarily flavonoids, namely kaempferol, quercetin, apigenin, luteolin, galangin, etc., then the phenolic acids and also phenolic acids derivatives. Polyphenols are heavily involved in influencing honey's properties. They are accountable for the anti-oxidant, anti-inflammatory and anti-angiogenic features of honey.

In addition, their impact on appearance can be seen in dark colored honeys, which have a higher amount of phenolic acids derivatives in contrast to the light ones, which in turn have more flavonoids.

Honey may additionally undergo an unwanted fermentation phenomenon, as it naturally possesses osmotolerant yeasts. That happens particularly in the case of a high moisture content of the honey. For that reason, when the yeast count is above 20 %, there is an increased risk of fermentation. Among the honeys with a significant yeast count are sunflower, rape, and tropical countries honeys.

Besides, pesticides, heavy metals, antibiotics and other environmental hazards can end up in honey. There are also toxic alkaloids in the nectar from some plants, although honey poisoning represents a rare event.

Concerning the microbial content, it should not be forgotten that honey is a highly dense sugar suspension. In this environment, because of the high osmotic pressure, microbes cannot find suitable growth conditions. Despite that, there are some bacteria which live in honey, yet the majority is harmless for humans. An exception is Clostridium botulinum, whose spores may land in the honey, and theoretically can develop the toxin in the body of infants. Such events have occurred very rarely. Nevertheless, in the US and the UK, health authorities advise not to give honey to infants. On the other hand, it should be pointed that these spores may be found in any natural food, and that mortality is actually very low in infant botulism, notwithstanding the severity of the disease.

In that concerning conservation, honey is quite fit to be stored as such over long periods of time. However, in order to preserve its properties as much as possible, honey must be kept in opaque, tightly sealed containers and in a cool atmosphere (between +4 and -10°C). That way, light will not break down the enzymes contained within.

Finally, one more mention about adulteration, which means a sort of "watering down" of honey through the mixing in of various syrups, sugars or other substances, so that honey acquires a new flavor, modifies its viscosity, does not crystallize or simply becomes cheaper to obtain. Such practices can be uncovered in case of corn syrup and cane sugar by using isotopic ratio mass spectrometry.

So, in the end, a truly pure honey signifies a honey free of any addition, be it sweeteners, water, flour, etc.

Classification of Honey

Ordering by floral source

This categorization refers to the origin of the nectar from which honey is obtained.

Thus, a monofloral honey comes mainly from one type of flower. This provenance will show in the specific flavor and color of the resulting honey. Examples of such honeys are those from acacia, lavender, thyme etc.

On the other extreme, we find the polyfloral honey (wildflower honey), based on the nectar from many types of flowers. In these honeys, there are variable mixtures of flavor and aroma.

Blended honey is a combination of different types of honey and represents most of the commercialized honey.

There is also a particular type of honey, called honeydew honey, characterized by a dark brown color and a stewed-fruit fragrance. In this case, the honey is produced from the sweet secretions of aphids (plant-sap sucking insects) and not from nectar. Pine honey from Greece is an example of honeydew honey.

Systematization by processing and packaging

As honey is commercialized in many forms, there is also a classification by processing and packaging, and the various types are succinctly described underneath.

Raw honey represents the real beehive honey, without processing, and may contain some pollen and wax.

Strained honey resembles raw honey in the pollen content, however, wax and other defects were cleared away by passing it through a mesh.

Filtered honey underwent a more advanced filtering process. Almost all particles were removed from suspension, and it was further subjected to a heating process (about 70°C).

Granulated or candied honey is a crystallized honey.

Pasteurized honey is considered a honey without yeast and a delayed crystallization, although enzymes activity may also be affected because of the heating. There are some changes in color, fragrance and taste, too.

Ultrasonicated honey is also a honey without viable yeasts, following ultrasonication. This process hinders further crystallization, too, but in contrast to pasteurization, the heating doesn't exceed 35°C.

Creamed honey or honey fondant is processed in such a way that it results a high number of tiny crystals, which prevent further crystallization and render a smoother honey.

Comb honey comes in chunks of cut-out wax combs.

When the comb honey is packed in recipients with liquid honey, the result is called *chunk honey*.

The latter two types of honey involve no processing, and they therefore preserve the honey's features, perhaps to the fullest extent.

How to buy quality honey

The very first thing people should know when it comes to obtaining good honey is that they cannot get it from a supermarket shelf. Likewise, they should not venture to acquire it from beekeepers they have no information about at all. And forget about honey produced by bee stocks based in industrial environments.

A truly pure honey should be sought in the country, in remote areas, as far away as possible from any pollution. The reason for this arises from the fact that only such surroundings make strong bee families, able to create honey with a higher biological value.

Unfortunately, there is no empiric method to establish the honey's degree of purity. The only reliable way to ascertain that is through complex laboratories, through the diastatic enzyme level, and HMF (the product resulted from fructose decay), among other methods.

As the value of the former parameter depends on the bee family, on their areal, as well as on honey processing ways, honey's maturity, its storage conditions and so on, it results a great variability of the honey quality. For example, one of the most valuable types of honey, the Siberian honey, reaches a value of over 50 points, even up to 65. At the other end of the spectrum, the honey produced by a weak bee family in an area heavily loaded with pesticides may measure only up to 9 points.

In conclusion, in order to benefit the most from the wonderful and unique qualities of this natural gold, aim for a raw honey.

Honey's Healing Features

As briefly depicted in the history chapter, honey has been extensively used for its healing effects. So, in the following section, we will dive a bit more in the ocean of features and therapeutic uses of the earth's gold.

But, before that, one more note: for the time being, we discuss only honey, as other bees' products (pollen, propolis, royal jelly, bee venom, podmore, beeswax and beehive air) are intended to make the content of the rest of this book series. Hopefully, you'll enjoy the ride.

First of all, honey stood out because of its antimicrobial characteristics. That is antibacterial, antiviral, antiparasitic, and antifungal features, and as such, it was also called a natural antibiotic. Honey's activity against bacteria was proven on many pathogenic strains, and underneath are listed a few examples:

- *Helicobacter pylori* - involved in stomach and duodenal ulcers;
- *Staphylococcus aureus* - responsible for many skin infections such as abscesses, wound infections, boils, impetigo, carbuncles;

- *Escherichia coli* - the cause of a wide range of various system infections, for example urinary infections, bowel infections (diarrhoea), wound infections, septicaemia etc.;

- *Pseudomonas aeruginosa* - the culprit in wound infections, urinary infections etc.;

- *Klebsiella pneumoniae* - responsible for a form of pneumonia;

- *Mycobacterium tuberculosis* - well known bacteria causing the main type of tuberculosis

And the list continues.

As mentioned above, honey has also antiviral and antiparasitic activity. It has been shown that honey inhibits *Rubella virus* - responsible for the rubella, *Echinococcus* - a parasite of tapeworm type, causing an infection named hydatid disease or echinococcosis, and *Leishmania* - a protozoan parasite, involved in leishmaniases.

Likewise, studies showed honey has a topical antifungal action against *Candida sp.* (cause of oral, gastro-intestinal and vaginal candidiasis), *Rhodotorula sp.* (opportunistic yeasts, agents of many diseases in humans, such as skin, ocular, prosthetic joint, peritoneal, and meningeal infections), etc.

It is worth noting that there are many intrinsic factors enabling honey to fight against these pathogens. Thus, the enzymes catalase and glucose oxidase exhibit both a hydrogen peroxide production capacity, a really powerful germ killer.

Antimicrobial activities are also displayed by other substances present in honey, by flavonoids, aromatic acids etc. Furthermore, honey viscosity (low water content), as well as its low pH play a substantial role in germs' break down. Moreover, this antimicrobial characteristic depends on the honey's floral source.

As indicated in various studies, honey has an intrinsic anti-oxidant capacity which plays a significant role in preventing aging and the degenerative, chronic diseases associated with it: cardio-vascular diseases, Alzheimer's disease and other brain dysfunctions, diabetes mellitus, cancer and immune-system downfall, cataracts, etc.

This effect stems from its content in phenolic compounds, including flavonoids (for instance carotenoid derivatives), phenolic acids, enzymes, namely catalase and glucose oxidase, organic acids, amino acids, proteins, vitamin C, etc.

Besides, research pointed to the direct anti-inflammatory effect of honey. Thus, in skin lesions without bacterial infection, it was observed such an action by the topical application of honey.

It seems that honey intake is as efficient in colitis subjects as prednisolone, a corticosteroid with powerful anti-inflammatory action. According to some studies, this effect is a consequence of hindering free radical production in inflamed tissues, as well as diminishing particular inflammation mediators (tromboxane B2, prostaglandins).

Similarly, this wonderful mixture is a known bio-stimulator, because of its content of various vitamins, anti-oxidants, and minerals (magnesium, iron, copper, selenium, manganese and others). As a result, by regular consumption, honey boosts immune system, increases leucocytes

(WBC), and probably can subdue pollen hypersensitivity, too.

Likewise, many studies in animals imply not only a relevant anti-mutagenic effect of honey (i.e. inhibits the alteration of the genetic material by particular mutagenic factors), but also a significant immunoprotective and anti-metastatic activity. Thus, oral intake of honey in cases of mammary carcinoma and colon adenocarcinoma in mice had shown an inhibitory effect on metastasis spreading, which statistically is significant.

In any event, considering honey's effect on immunity, as well as its antimicrobial and anti-inflammatory properties, it is easy to understand its good functioning in various infections of different body systems.

In respiratory infections, starting with the common cold, continuing with sinusitis, sore throat, bronchitis and pneumonia, honey is especially good due to the already mentioned features, as well as to its expectorant and soothing capacities for sore throat. Similarly, as it also has a beneficial effect on allergies, honey induces an overall positive outcome in asthma.

Likewise, honey leads to a positive result in urinary infections, through its antimicrobial and anti-inflammatory properties. Moreover, its composition has beneficial effects in kidney stones and prostate enlargement.

Furthermore, this powerful food helps with the overall digestive health. Its actions start in the mouth, where it leads to healing and improvement of the lining, in conditions such as stomatitis, oral or labial herpes, oral candidiasis, etc. Oral ulcers are also successfully healed. And again, it sooths toothache and fights cavities and plaque.

In heartburn (gastro-esophageal reflux disease - GERD), honey use was proved advantageous, both due to the coating of the esophagus lining, with beneficial local effects, and the healing of associated stomach diseases (such as gastritis and peptic ulcers).

Identically, in stomach and small bowel it covers the lining and the ulcers, promoting their healing. In fact, it also inhibits powerfully the growth of *Helicobacter pylori*, considered as the cause of many gastritis and peptic ulcers.

According to research results, there are many mechanisms involved in these effects: its anti-oxidant activity, the protection of key anti-oxidant factors in the gastric tissue (such as glutathione), and the promotion of intra-gastric nitric oxide formation, substance which boosts lining formation. Regular honey consumption leads to diminished gastric acid secretion, with positive outcomes in peptic ulcer, as showed in a study.

In addition, honey fights indigestion, helps with the growth of stomach beneficial bacteria, and lends a hand in getting rid of intestinal parasites. Being also a great laxative, honey works beautifully in constipation. Last, but not least, it is a fantastic food, full of nutrients, vitamins and trace elements.

A diet or preparates with honey are good in preventing and treating cardio-vascular diseases, and, again, that is achieved through its anti-inflammatory and anti-oxidant activity. Thus, studies revealed that honey diminishes the levels of LDL-cholesterol and triglycerides in blood, all of these being well-known risk factors in cardio-vascular conditions. Moreover, its effects lead to a reduction of platelet aggregation and blood coagulation. Finally, honey is reputed to be a good tonic for heart, and, according to an in vitro study in animals, long-term honey intake has protective effects against heart-attacks and palpitations.

Honey may also help with obesity, perhaps when entirely replacing the sugar intake. It seems that honey's fructose has a nutritional benefit through lowering triglycerides in blood, in contrast with sucrose, which increases them. It was also proved that it has a positive effect in regulation of blood sugar levels.

Moreover, honey appears to regulate appetite hormones, leading to lower food intake in obesity. Conversely, in anorexia it seems to increase appetite. The overall benefit of honey in anorexia stems also from the high nutritional values of its various components.

Besides, research evidence indicates honey's positive effects on endocrine system. For instance, in diabetic patients, honey used as a sweetener produced a notably lower increase in blood glucose contrasted with sucrose or glucose. It also regulates blood sugar, promotes insulin secretion, and ameliorates the lipid profile. All these findings indicate that honey may be used as a sweetener at least in type 2 diabetes.

Likewise, honey may play the role of hormone replacement therapy in menopause, as it acts towards increasing bone density, protecting against uterine atrophy and high body weight. Also, menopausal symptoms are alleviated by daily consumption of honey.

Furthermore, studies pinpointed to the therapeutic role of honey in anemia. Daily doses of honey led to normal blood values of hemoglobin.

Honey's favorable actions reach to the neuropsychiatric sphere. Through its calmative properties, it fights insomnia and sooths anxiety disorders. It also has regenerative and neuroprotective features. Thus, in Ayurveda, honey is used to increase longevity and better focusing and memory. Also, it helps in dementia and Alzheimer's disease, through improvement and prevention of cognitive impairment, as showed in a 5-year pilot study.

As already mentioned, because of its content in anti-oxidants, flavonoids and others, honey has anti-cancer properties, as shown in studies re this topic. Moreover, administered in patients undergoing chemo- and radiotherapy, it displayed beneficial effects, decreasing the side-effects commonly associated with these treatments: mucositis (inflammation of the linings), weight-loss, and neutropenia (low number of white blood cells).

Again, Ayurveda has been recommending honey for the treatment of various eye conditions (conjunctivitis, keratitis, blepharitis, corneal ulcers). Similarly, in European eastern countries, eye infections and burns have been successfully healed with honey. The curing effects are doubtlessly due to honey's antimicrobial and anti-inflammatory features.

And that's also the reason why honey is good at treating acne and various wounds - bed sores, abrasions, burns, skin infections, and ulcers. Additionally, as a great moisturizer, with regenerative, anti-dandruff and nourishing properties, honey is one of the best classical treatments for beautiful skin and hair.

Overall, honey consumption reduces fatigue, offers an energy boost, and ameliorates athlete's performance. In fact, it is one of the most effective energizers in nature.

Finally, it should be highlighted that combining honey with fruits, vegetables or medicinal herbs leads to synergistic effects, amplifying the benefits of each component.

However, particular attention should be paid to adverse effects and contraindications, as well as in case of multiple conditions and their respective treatments. We advocate the unfolding of treatments with honey under medical supervision.

Final Thoughts:

- Honey should be always taken in lukewarm beverages (up to 40°C), so that its components are not damaged.

- Before starting a treatment, seek medical advice.

- In order to obtain benefits, honey should be taken daily over at least 2 weeks. There are some advocating a minimum daily honey consumption for one and a half months.

- Normally, sweeteners should not exceed 25 grams per day. Therefore, when beginning a treatment with honey, avoid other sugars.

- In adults, the intake of 50 to 80, with a maximum of 100 grams honey per day is recommended, or apply the general formula (adults and infants) 1 g honey per kg weight.

- Don't give honey to children under 1 year.

Part 2 - Honey Therapy

Chapter 4

Respiratory diseases

Asthma

Asthma is a long-term condition that leads to narrowing and inflammation of the airways, as well as an excessive mucus production. The symptoms are different from one person to another, may be sporadic or often, or may occur only in particular circumstances: triggered by inhalant substances (allergy-induced asthma), by cold and dry air (exercise-induced asthma), and by irritants in the work environment (occupational asthma). Asthma occurs especially in children.

Symptoms:

- wheezing (whistling while breathing) - the major symptom of asthma. The patient has repeating episodes of wheezing.
- shortness of breath
- coughing - often during night or in the morning
- chest tightness

Seek medical advice when the above-mentioned symptomatology occurs or when asthma symptoms are more often and distressing, with an increased breathing difficulty, or when requiring more frequent use of the inhaler.

Risk factors:

- smoking or exposure to smoke
- exposure to inhalant pollutants and occupational triggers
- obesity
- associated allergic conditions
- relatives with asthma

Recipe 1 - Honey and Water

Difficulty: +; Time: 2-3 minutes;

Ingredients:
- 1 1/2 teaspoon honey
- Water or tea

Preparation: Mix thoroughly honey with lukewarm water or tea.

How to take it: Three times a day, half an hour before meal.

Tips:
- Use organic raw honey
- Use regularly for better effects

Precautions:
- Do not use if you are allergic to any ingredient
- Contact your doctor with any questions or concerns

Disclaimer: This does not replace medical advice. Check With Your Doctor for symptoms or worsening of condition.

Recipe 2 - Honey and Milk

Difficulty: +; Time: 2 - 3 minutes;

Ingredients:

- 1 1/2 teaspoon honey
- 1 glass of milk

Preparation: Mix honey with lukewarm milk.

How to take it: Three times a day, half an hour before meal.

Tips:

- Use organic raw honey and milk.
- Use regularly for better effects

Precautions:

- Do not use if you are allergic to any ingredient
- Do not use if you have lactose intolerance
- Contact your doctor with any questions or concerns

Disclaimer: This does not replace medical advice. Check With Your Doctor for symptoms or worsening of condition.

Recipe 3 - Honey and Lemon

Difficulty: +; Time: 2 - 3 minutes;

Ingredients:

- 1 1/2 teaspoon honey
- Juice from half a lemon
- Water or tea

Preparation: Mix thoroughly honey with lemon juice and lukewarm water or tea.

How to take it: Three times a day, half an hour before meal.

Tips:

- Lemon properties: contains vitamins (A, B complex, C, E), minerals (calcium, magnesium, potassium, copper, manganese, zinc, iron), flavonoids (naringin, naringenin, hesperetin, alfa- and beta-carotenes, lutein, zeaxanthin, beta-cryptoxanthin, tannins), terpenes, citric acid, fibers; anti-oxidant, anti-inflammatory, anti-bacterial, antifungal, antiseptic, immune system booster.

- Lemon beneficial effects: dyspepsia, constipation, respiratory infections, asthma, rheumatism, arthritis, lowers blood pressure, helps with weight-loss, anti-cancer, acne, eczema, burns.
- Use organic raw honey and lemon.
- Use regularly for better effects

Precautions:

- Lemon may cause photosensitivity when used on skin
- Do not use if you are allergic to any ingredient
- Take after meal in case of stomach ulcer
- Contact your doctor with any questions or concerns

Disclaimer: This does not replace medical advice. Check With Your Doctor for symptoms or worsening of condition.

Recipe 4 - Honey and Grapefruit Juice

Difficulty: +; Time: 2-3 minutes;

Ingredients:

- 1 tablespoon honey
- 1 glass of grapefruit juice

Preparation: Mix honey with juice.

How to take it: In the morning, 30 minutes before meal.

Tips:

- Grapefruit properties: contains vitamins (A, B complex, C, D, E), minerals (copper, potassium, calcium, magnesium, phosphorous, zinc), limonoids (limonin glucosyde), flavonoids (naringenin, alpha- and beta-carotens, lutein, zeaxanthin), pectin, fats, fibers; anti-oxidant, boosts immunity, lowers cholesterol and triglycerides, decreases insulin resistance, lowers blood pressure, anti-cancer.
- Grapefruit beneficial effects: infections, fatigue, cardio-vascular diseases, degenerative diseases (Alzheimer's disease, Parkinson disease),

prevents kidney stones, helps with digestion, constipation, flatulence, helps with weight-loss.
- Use organic raw honey and grapefruit.
- Use regularly for better effects

Precautions:

- Grapefruit has many interactions with drugs: anticoagulants (blood thinners), benzodiazepines, immunosuppressants, Indinavir, carbamazepine (anti-convulsives), some statins, most calcium channel blockers. Ask your doctor before starting a cure!!!
- Do not use if you are allergic to any ingredient
- Contact your doctor with any questions or concerns

Disclaimer: This does not replace medical advice. Check With Your Doctor for symptoms or worsening of condition.

Recipe 5 - Honey and Cinnamon

Difficulty: +; Time: 2 - 3 minutes;

Ingredients:

- 1 tablespoon honey
- 1/3 teaspoon cinnamon
- water or tea

Preparation: Mix thoroughly honey and cinnamon with lukewarm water or tea.

How to take it: In the morning, 30 minutes before meal or at bed time.

Tips:

- Cinnamon properties: contains vitamins (A, B complex, C), minerals (calcium, iron, manganese, phosphorous), essential oils (cinnamaldehyde, cinnamyl alcohol, cinnamyl acetate), flavonoids (alpha- and beta-carotens, lutein, zeaxanthin, cryptoxanthin, lycopene); anti-oxidant, anti-inflammatory, antimicrobial, antifungal, analgesic, anti-spastic, anti-parasites, haemostatic, peripheral vasodilator, lowers cholesterol, reduces stress and fatigue, promotes healing, anti-cancer.

- Cinnamon beneficial effects: infections (respiratory, gynecological: leucorrhea, vaginitis; digestive: gingivitis, mouth ulcers, enterocolitis, amoebiasis), dyspepsia, GERD, gastritis, peptic ulcer, asthenia, depression, Alzheimer, regulates menstruation, eczema, helps with weight-loss.
- Use organic raw honey and cinnamon.
- Use regularly for better effects

Precautions:

- Not to be used in pregnancy and in breast-feeding women
- Do not use if you are allergic to any ingredient
- Contact your doctor with any questions or concerns

Disclaimer: This does not replace medical advice. Check With Your Doctor for symptoms or worsening of condition.

Bronchitis

The acute form of bronchitis (chest cold) is a short term inflammatory condition usually caused by a viral infection of the bronchi (lung airways), whereas in the chronic bronchitis there is a productive cough which lasts at least 3 months per year, over 2 years. The majority of those with chronic bronchitis have COPD (chronic obstructive pulmonary disease).

Symptoms in acute bronchitis:

- productive cough - the most common symptom
- wheezing (whistling while breathing)
- shortness of breath
- fever
- chest discomfort

Symptoms in chronic bronchitis:

- productive cough - especially in the morning
- wheezing (whistling while breathing)
- shortness of breath

Seek medical advice when coughing more than 3 weeks, when the cough is associated with high fever, shortness of breath or wheezing, when it interferes with the sleep, or there is a discolored or bloody flegma

Risk factors:

- smoking
- occupational exposure to irritants
- severe heartburn (gastric reflux) may irritate the throat and may predispose to bronchitis
- incompetent or weak immune system such as during another acute or chronic disease, or in particular age groups (infants, young children and elderly)

Recipe 6 - Honey and Turmeric

Difficulty: +; Time: 2 - 3 minutes;

Ingredients:

- 1 tablespoon honey
- 1 teaspoon turmeric powder

Preparation: Mix the honey with turmeric powder.

How to take it: In the morning, 30 minutes before meal.

Tips:

- Turmeric properties: vitamins (B complex, C, E, K), minerals (potassium, calcium, magnesium, copper, phosphorous, zinc, iron, selenium, manganese), curcuminoids (curcumin, demethoxycurcumin), volatile oils (turmerone, zingiberene, atlantone), resins, proteins, sugars; anti-inflammatory, mood improvement, blood thinning, lowers cholesterol, modulation of the immune response, painkiller, in Type 2 Diabetes reduces blood sugar and diminishes insulin resistance, anti-cancer.

- Turmeric beneficial effects: infections, Alzheimer's disease, depression, arthritis, inflammatory digestive tract diseases, cardio-vascular diseases, obesity, psoriasis, autoimmune diseases (lupus, rheumatoid arthritis, etc.).
- Use organic raw honey and turmeric.
- Use regularly for better effects

Precautions:

- Turmeric contraindications: pregnant women, during menstruation. Side-Effects: nausea and diarrhea, lower blood pressure, higher bleeding risk (especially combined with anticoagulants). If you are on anticoagulants (blood thinners), ask your doctor before starting a cure!!!
- Do not use if you are allergic to any ingredient
- Contact your doctor with any questions or concerns

Disclaimer: This does not replace medical advice. Check With Your Doctor for symptoms or worsening of condition.

Recipe 7 - Honey, Lemon and Black Radish

Difficulty: +; Time: 5 minutes;

Ingredients:

- 1 tablespoon honey
- 1 teaspoon lemon juice
- 1 black radish

Preparation: Use a juicer or blender to extract radish juice. Mix honey with radish and lemon juice.

How to take it: Once per day, in the morning before breakfast or at bed time.

Tips:

- Lemon properties: contains vitamins (A, B complex, C, E), minerals (calcium, magnesium, potassium, copper, manganese, zinc, iron), flavonoids (naringin, naringenin, hesperetin, alfa- and beta-carotenes, lutein, zeaxanthin, beta-cryptoxanthin, tannins), terpenes, citric acid, fibers; anti-oxidant, anti-inflammatory, anti-bacterial, antifungal, antiseptic, immune system booster.

- Lemon beneficial effects: dyspepsia, constipation, respiratory infections, asthma, rheumatism, arthritis, lowers blood pressure, helps with weight-loss, anti-cancer, acne, eczema, burns.
- Black radish properties: contains vitamins (C, B complex), minerals (calcium, magnesium, copper, iron), indoles, flavonoids (zeaxanthin, lutein, beta-carotens, anthocyanins), high fiber content; expectorant, anti-congestive, bactericidal, disinfectant, antioxidant, diuretic, lowers body fever, lowers blood pressure, decreases blood sugar, anti-cancer.
- Black radish beneficial effects: respiratory infections (asthma, bronchitis, pneumonia convalescence, sinusitis and sore throats), high blood pressure, constipation, weight loss, diabetes, many types of cancers, in skin disorders.
- Use organic raw honey, lemon and black radish
- Use regularly for better effects

Precautions:

- Lemon may cause photosensitivity when used on skin
- Do not use if you are allergic to any ingredient
- Contact your doctor with any questions or concerns

Disclaimer: This does not replace medical advice. Check With Your Doctor for symptoms or worsening of condition.

Recipe 8 - Honey and Apple Cider Vinegar

Difficulty: +; Time: 2-3 minutes;

Ingredients:

- 1 tablespoon honey
- 1 tablespoon of apple cider vinegar
- 1 glass with water

Preparation: Mix honey with water and apple cider vinegar.

How to take it: Drink it at bed time.

Tips:

- Apple cider vinegar properties: contains vitamins (B complex, C, pantothenic acid), minerals (calcium, potassium, sodium, iron, phosphorus), acetic acid, malic acid, pectin, polyphenols (flavonols, flavanols, tannins, anthocyanins, dihydrochalcones, hydroxycinnamic acids); boosts immunity, anti-microbial, anti-inflammatory, antioxidant, lowers cholesterol, lowers blood sugar, acts as anti-acid.
- Apple cider vinegar beneficial effects: in infections (sinusitis, sore throat, asthma, other res-

piratory infections, urinary tract infections, etc), allergies, arthritis, gout, cardiovascular diseases, improves digestion, prevents constipation, helps with weight loss, in skin conditions (acne, eczema).
- Use organic raw honey and apple cider vinegar.
- Use regularly for better effects

Precautions:

- Do not use if you are allergic to any ingredient
- Contact your doctor with any questions or concerns

Disclaimer: This does not replace medical advice. Check With Your Doctor for symptoms or worsening of condition.

Recipe 9 - Honey and Thyme

Difficulty: +; Time: 30 minutes;

Ingredients:
- 1 teaspoon honey
- 1 teaspoon Thyme
- 1 glass water

Preparation: Prepare an infusion with Thyme and leave it to cool. Mix honey with the infusion.

How to take it: 3 times daily, 30 minutes before meals.

Tips:

• Thyme properties: contains vitamins (A, B complex, C), minerals (copper, iron, manganese, calcium, magnesium), flavonoids (thymonin, apigenin, luteolin, naringenin), carvacrol, fibers; antimicrobial, antifungal, anti-oxidant, boosts immunity, lowers cholesterol, helps with cough, diuretic, stimulates appetite, improves mood.

• Thyme beneficial effects: respiratory infections (asthma, cold, bronchitis), digestive problems (dyspepsia, flatulence, biliary dyskinesia),

skin infections, lowers blood pressure, anorexia, depression, rheumatism, gout.
- Use organic raw honey and thyme.
- Use regularly for better effects

Precautions:

- Thyme: avoid in pregnancy and breast-feeding.
- Do not use if you are allergic to any ingredient
- Contact your doctor with any questions or concerns

Disclaimer: This does not replace medical advice. Check With Your Doctor for symptoms or worsening of condition.

Recipe 10 - Honey and Cloves

Difficulty: +; Time: 30 minutes;

Ingredients:

- 1 tablespoon honey
- 3-4 cloves
- 1 glass water

Preparation: Prepare an infusion with cloves and leave it to cool. Mix honey with the infusion.

How to take it: In the morning, 30 minutes before meal and at bed time.

Tips:

- Cloves properties: contain vitamins (A, B complex, C, K), minerals (calcium, magnesium, copper, iron, manganese, selenium, zinc, phosphorous), flavonoids (rhamnetin, eugenin, eugenitin, kaempferol, beta-carotene, tannins such as methyl salicylate, gallotannic acid), essential oils (acetyl eugenol, vanillin, maslinic acid, β-caryophyllene), triterpenoids (campesterol, stigmasterol, oleanolic acid); anti-oxidant, anti-inflammatory, antiseptic, anti-bacterial, fight against intestinal parasites, analgesic, boost the immune system, lower blood

sugar, anti-nausea, dyspepsia, anti-flatulent, reduce stress, anti-cancer.
- Cloves beneficial effects: asthma, respiratory infections, sinusitis, rheumatism, gout, improve digestion, acne, diabetes.
- Use organic raw honey and cloves.
- Use regularly for better effects

Precautions:

- Cloves contraindications: avoid in pregnancy, stomach ulcers or if under treatment with anticoagulants. If you are on anticoagulants (blood thinners), ask your doctor before starting a cure!!!
- Do not use if you are allergic to any ingredient
- Contact your doctor with any questions or concerns

Disclaimer: This does not replace medical advice. Check With Your Doctor for symptoms or worsening of condition.

Acute Pharyngitis

Pharyngitis is an upper respiratory tract infection in which the back of the throat is especially afflicted. Subtypes include common cold and tonsillitis.

Common Cold (Nasopharyngitis)

Common cold or the cold is a viral infection of the upper airways that affects the nose, the sinuses and the throat.

Symptoms of common cold:

- cough and sneezing
- runny nose
- sore throat
- fever
- headache

Seek medical advice if high fever, recurrent or more than 5-day fever, severe sore throat and shortness of breath.

Risk factors:

- certain group ages (children up to 6 years old and the elderly)
- smoking
- chronic illness
- weak immune system
- season (fall and winter)
- spending time in large groups

Recipe 11 - Honey and Sunflower Seed Powder

Difficulty: +; Time: 2-3 minutes;

Ingredients:

- 1 tablespoon honey
- 1 teaspoon sunflower seeds powder

Preparation: Mix honey with sunflower seeds powder.

How to take it: In the morning, 30 minutes before meal and in the evening.

Tips:

- Sunflower seeds properties: contain vitamins (B complex, E), minerals (magnesium, phosphorous, copper, selenium, manganese, zinc, iron, potassium), phytosterols, flavonoids (alpha- and beta-carotene); anti-oxidant, anti-inflammatory, decrease cholesterol, lower blood pressure, lower blood sugar, anti-cancer.
- Sunflower seeds beneficial effects: respiratory infections, asthma, high blood pressure, diabetes, degenerative disorders (Parkinson disease, Alzheimer's disease), depression, anxiety, hormonal regulation (especially thyroid), osteoporosis.

- Use organic raw honey and sunflower seeds.
- Use regularly for better effects

Precautions:

- Do not use if you are allergic to any ingredient
- Contact your doctor with any questions or concerns

Disclaimer: This does not replace medical advice. Check With Your Doctor for symptoms or worsening of condition.

Recipe 12 - Honey, Fenugreek and Ginger

Difficulty: +; Time: 3 minutes (requires overnight soaking of the fenugreek seeds);

Ingredients:

- 1 tablespoon honey
- 1 teaspoon ginger juice
- 1 1/2 teaspoon fenugreek seeds
- 1 glass water

Preparation: Mix seeds with water and let them soak overnight. In the morning, mix them with honey and ginger juice.

How to take it: 30 minutes before meals, in the morning and at bed time.

Tips:

- Ginger properties: contains vitamins (B complex, C, E), minerals (calcium, magnesium, phosphorous, potassium, sodium, zinc, iron), gingerols, zingerone, shogaols (volatile oils), beta-carotene, capsaicin, caffeic acid, curcumin, salicylate; anti-oxidant, anti-inflammatory, antibacterial, antifungal, analgesic, anti-nausea, lowers cholesterol, choleretic, anti-cancer.

- Ginger beneficial effects: respiratory infections, asthma, heart disease, GERD, stomach ulcer, diabetes prevention and therapy, weight loss.
- Fenugreek seeds properties: contain vitamins (B complex), minerals (magnesium, manganese, phosphorous, iron, copper, calcium), choline, tigogenin, trigonelline diosgenin, neotigogens, yamogenin, gitogenin, tannins, mucilage, pectins, saponins, fibers, non-starch polysaccharides; anti-inflammatory, emollient, lower cholesterol and triglycerides, anti-cancer, stimulate insulin release, increase appetite.
- Fenugreek seeds beneficial effects: respiratory infections, asthma, mouth ulcers, arthritis, gout, eating disorders, improve muscular performance, eczema, wounds, constipation, hemorrhoids.
- Use organic raw honey, fenugreek and ginger.
- Use regularly for better effects

Precautions:

- Ginger should be avoided in pregnancy and breastfeeding. It may cause blood thinning. If you are on anticoagulants (blood thinners), ask your doctor before starting a cure!!! Precaution is advised when using blood pressure medication.
- Fenugreek seeds may cause blood thinning. If you are on anticoagulants (blood thinners), ask your doctor before starting a cure!!! They may also cause flatulence and diarrhea, applied on skin may induce irritation.

- Do not use if you are allergic to any ingredient
- Contact your doctor with any questions or concerns

Disclaimer: This does not replace medical advice. Check With Your Doctor for symptoms or worsening of condition.

Recipe 13 - Honey, Ginger and Black Pepper

Difficulty: +; Time: 2-3 minutes;

Ingredients:

- 1 tablespoon honey
- 1 teaspoon minced ginger
- 1 pinch black pepper

Preparation: Mix honey with ginger and black pepper.

How to take it: In the morning, 30 minutes before meal.

Tips:

- Ginger properties: contains vitamins (B complex, C, E), minerals (calcium, magnesium, phosphorous, potassium, sodium, zinc, iron), gingerols, zingerone, shogaols (volatile oils), beta-carotene, capsaicin, caffeic acid, curcumin, salicylate;

anti-oxidant, anti-inflammatory, antibacterial, antifungal, analgesic, anti-nausea, lowers cholesterol, choleretic, anti-cancer.
- Ginger beneficial effects: respiratory infections, asthma, heart disease, GERD, stomach ulcer, diabetes prevention and therapy, weight loss.
- Black pepper properties: contains vitamins (A, B complex, C, E, K), choline, minerals (calcium, magnesium, manganese, copper, iron, zinc), piperine (essential oil), monoterpenes (pinene, sabinene, mercene, limonene, terpenene), flavonoids (carotenes, lycopene, zea-xanthin, cryptoxanthin); anti-oxidant, anti-inflammatory, anti-bacterial, analgesic, carminative, anti-flatulent.
- Black pepper beneficial effects: respiratory infections, asthma, weight loss, constipation, anemia, gastric and duodenal ulcers, ear- and toothaches, heart disease, cognitive impairment (Alzheimer's disease, dementia), and helps with vitiligo.
- Use organic raw honey, ginger and black pepper.
- Use regularly for better effects

Precautions:

- Ginger should be avoided in pregnancy and breastfeeding. It may cause blood thinning. If you are on anticoagulants (blood thinners), ask your doctor before starting a cure!!! Precaution is advised when using blood pressure medication.

- Black pepper may cause skin irritation after direct application; consumed in large amounts in pregnancy may induce miscarriage, and high intake is not recommended in ulcers.
- Do not use if you are allergic to any ingredient
- Contact your doctor with any questions or concerns

Disclaimer: This does not replace medical advice. Check With Your Doctor for symptoms or worsening of condition.

Recipe 14 - Honey, Lemon and Ginger

Difficulty: +; Time 30 minutes;

Ingredients:

- 1 tablespoon honey
- 1 tablespoon grated ginger
- juice from 1/2 lemon
- 1 glass of water

Preparation: Infused grated ginger in boiling water, leave to cool 20 minutes. Then, mix in honey and lemon juice.

How to take it: In the morning, 30 minutes before meal.

Tips:

- Lemon properties: contains vitamins (A, B complex, C, E), minerals (calcium, magnesium, potassium, copper, manganese, zinc, iron), flavonoids (naringin, naringenin, hesperetin, alfa- and beta-carotenes, lutein, zeaxanthin, beta-cryptoxanthin, tannins), terpenes, citric acid, fibers; anti-oxidant, anti-inflammatory, anti-bacterial, antifungal, antiseptic, immune system booster.

- Lemon beneficial effects: dyspepsia, constipation, respiratory infections, asthma, rheumatism, arthritis, lowers blood pressure, helps with weight-loss, anti-cancer, acne, eczema, burns.
- Ginger properties: contains vitamins (B complex, C, E), minerals (calcium, magnesium, phosphorous, potassium, sodium, zinc, iron), gingerols, zingerone, shogaols (volatile oils), beta-carotene, capsaicin, caffeic acid, curcumin, salicylate; anti-oxidant, anti-inflammatory, antibacterial, antifungal, analgesic, anti-nausea, lowers cholesterol, choleretic, anti-cancer.
- Ginger beneficial effects: respiratory infections, asthma, heart disease, GERD, stomach ulcer, diabetes prevention and therapy, weight loss.
- Use organic raw honey, lemon and ginger.
- Use regularly for better effects

Precautions:

- Ginger should be avoided in pregnancy and breastfeeding. It may cause blood thinning. If you are on anticoagulants (blood thinners), ask your doctor before starting a cure!!! Precaution is advised when using blood pressure medication.
- Lemon may cause photosensitivity when used on skin
- Do not use if you are allergic to any ingredient
- Contact your doctor with any questions or concerns

Disclaimer: This does not replace medical advice. Check With Your Doctor for symptoms or worsening of condition.

Acute Tonsillitis (Sore Throat)

Acute tonsillitis is an infection of the tonsils, mostly of viral origin.

Symptoms:

- sore throat
- swollen tonsils
- fever
- difficulty swallowing
- swollen glands around the neck
- feeling unwell in general

Seek medical advice for persistent, over 1 or 2 days sore throat, in children, extreme fatigue, difficulty breathing and swallowing.

Risk factors:

- young age: bacterial tonsillitis in age group 5 to 15, viral tonsillitis in age group under 5 years
- exposure

Recipe 15 - Honey, Lemon and Red Onion

Difficulty: ++; Time: up to 60 minutes, requires overnight storage;

Ingredients:
- 2 tablespoons honey
- juice from 1/2 lemon
- 2 medium red onions
- 400 ml water

Preparation: Chop the onions and boil them in the water, so that the volume decreases to 1/3. Let the mixture cool, then add lemon juice and honey and stir well. Store overnight.

How to take it: 1 tablespoon 30 minutes before meals for adults. For children, the intake is only 1 teaspoon 30 minutes before meals.

Tips:
- Onion properties: contains vitamins (B complex, C, D), minerals (calcium, magnesium, potassium, copper, phosphorus, manganese), flavonoids (quercetin, fisetin, tannins, anthocyanins),

thiosulfinates, fiber; anti-oxidant, anti-inflammatory, decreases cholesterol, improves mood and lowers blood sugar, anti-cancer.
- Onion beneficial effects: prevention and improvement in heart diseases, respiratory infections, asthma, sinusitis, depression, improves sleep.
- Lemon properties: contains vitamins (A, B complex, C, E), minerals (calcium, magnesium, potassium, copper, manganese, zinc, iron), flavonoids (naringin, naringenin, hesperetin, alfa- and beta-carotenes, lutein, zeaxanthin, beta-cryptoxanthin, tannins), terpenes, citric acid, fibers; anti-oxidant, anti-inflammatory, anti-bacterial, antifungal, antiseptic, immune system booster.
- Lemon beneficial effects: dyspepsia, constipation, respiratory infections, asthma, rheumatism, arthritis, lowers blood pressure, helps with weight-loss, anti-cancer, acne, eczema, burns.
- Use organic raw honey, lemon and onion.
- Use regularly for better effects

Precautions:

- Red onion may cause bloating, in high amounts may interfere with blood thinning. If you are on anticoagulants (blood thinners), ask your doctor before starting a cure!!
- Lemon may cause photosensitivity when used on skin
- Do not use if you are allergic to any ingredient

- Contact your doctor with any questions or concerns

Disclaimer: This does not replace medical advice. Check With Your Doctor for symptoms or worsening of condition.

Recipe 16 - Honey and Indian Gooseberries (Alma)

Difficulty: +; Time: 2-3 minutes;

Ingredients:

- 1 tablespoon honey
- 1/2 teaspoon Indian gooseberries powder or 2 teaspoons crushed Indian gooseberries

Preparation: Mix honey with Indian gooseberries powder or with crushed ones.

How to take it: In the morning, 30 minutes before meal or at bed time.

Tips:

- Indian gooseberries properties: contain vitamins (A, B complex, C), minerals (calcium, magnesium, sodium, potassium, iron, copper, zinc, manganese), polyphenols such as flavones, phyllanemblin, phyllanemblinin A, punicafolin, flavonoids (anthocyanins, kampferol), gallic acid, ellagic acid, ellagitannins (punigluconin, emblicanin A and B, pedunculagin), high fiber content; antioxidant, anti-bacterial, anti-inflammatory, boost

immunity, lower cholesterol and blood sugar, increase calcium absorption, laxative, diuretic.
- Indian gooseberries beneficial effects: respiratory infections, asthma, urinary tract infections, arthritis, anemia, heart disease, diabetes, improve appetite, help with weight-loss and constipation.
- Use organic raw honey and gooseberries.
- Use regularly for better effects

Precautions:

- Indian gooseberries may interfere with blood thinning. If you are on anticoagulants (blood thinners), ask your doctor before starting a cure!!!
- Do not use if you are allergic to any ingredient
- Contact your doctor with any questions or concerns

Disclaimer: This does not replace medical advice. Check With Your Doctor for symptoms or worsening of condition.

Recipe 17 - Honey, Garlic and Olive Oil

Difficulty: +; Time: 5 minutes;

Ingredients:

- 1 tablespoon honey
- 1 teaspoon olive oil
- juice from 2-3 garlic cloves
- 1 glass water

Preparation: Mix honey with olive oil and garlic juice, then add 1 glass lukewarm water. Stir well.

How to take it: In the morning, 30 minutes before meal.

Tips:

- Garlic properties: contains vitamins (A, B complex, C, K), minerals (calcium, magnesium, iron, manganese, potassium, selenium, zinc, phosphorous), thiosulfinates (allicin, methyl allyl sulfinates), ajoenes, sulfides, sulfoxides (alliin, isoalliin, methiin, garlicins), flavonoids (beta-carotene, lutein, zeaxanthin); anti-bacterial, anti-viral, anti-fungal, anti-inflammatory, anti-oxidant, anti-platelet activity, decreases cholesterol, lowers blood sugar, lowers blood pressure.

- Garlic beneficial effects: heart diseases, high blood pressure, various cancers, respiratory infections, sinusitis, asthma, gastric and duodenal ulcers, especially associated with *Helicobacter pylori*, liver cirrhosis, osteoporosis, improves performance and reduces fatigue, detoxifies the body of heavy metals.
- Olive oil properties: contains vitamins (E, K), fatty acids (high content of oleic acid, omega-3, omega-6), flavonoids: flavonols (kaempferol, quercetin), flavones (luteolin, apigenin), anthocyanidins (peonidins, cyanidins), as well as tyrosols (tyrosol, hydroxytyrosol, oleuropein), secoiridoids (oleuropein), hydroxybenzoic acids (syringic acid, vanillic acid), hydroxycinnamic acids (coumaric acid, caffeic acid, ferulic acid, cinnamic acid), lignans (pinoresinol); lowers blood pressure, lowers cholesterol, anti-oxidant, antimicrobial (including *Helicobacter pylori*), anti-inflammatory, promotes bone formation.
- Olive oil beneficial effects: heart diseases, diabetes, osteoporosis, anti-cancer, respiratory infections, stomach and duodenal ulcer (especially associated with *Helicobacter pylori*), weight-loss.
- Use organic raw honey, garlic and olive oil.
- Use regularly for better effects

Precautions:

- Garlic: may lower Saquinavir levels and may interact with some anticoagulants and diabetes medication. If you are on anticoagulants (blood thinners), ask your doctor before starting a cure!!! May cause flatulence and nausea. Locally applied may lead to irritation, urticaria, anaphylaxis.
- Do not use if you are allergic to any ingredient
- Contact your doctor with any questions or concerns

Disclaimer: This does not replace medical advice. Check With Your Doctor for symptoms or worsening of condition.

Recipe 18 - Honey and Safflower

Difficulty: +; Time: 2-3 minutes;

Ingredients:

- 2 teaspoons honey
- 1/2 teaspoon safflower seed powder

Preparation: Mix honey with safflower seed powder.

How to take it: 30 minutes before meals, twice a day.

Tips:

- Safflower properties: contains vitamins (A, B complex), minerals (potassium, phosphorous, magnesium, calcium, zinc, iron, manganese, copper), fatty acids (oleic, linoleic), tracheloside (lignan glycoside), serotonin derivatives, alpha- and gamma tocopherol; anti-oxidant, lowers cholesterol, laxative, sedative, expectorant.
- Safflower beneficial effects: respiratory infections, asthma, cardiovascular diseases, osteoporosis, rheumatism, dyspepsia, constipation, helps with weight-loss.
- Use organic raw honey and safflower.

- Use regularly for better effects

Precautions:

- Safflower contraindications: in large amount, may impair blood clotting; interacts with blood thinning drugs (Aspirin, Diclofenac, Ibuprofen, Warfarin, Clopidogrel, and others). If you are on anticoagulant (blood thinners), ask your doctor before starting a cure!!!
- Do not use if you are allergic to any ingredient
- Contact your doctor with any questions or concerns

Disclaimer: This does not replace medical advice. Check With Your Doctor for symptoms or worsening of condition.

Recipe 19 - Honey, Bitter Gourd and Great Basil

Difficulty: +; Time: 10 minutes;

Ingredients:

- 1 tablespoon honey
- 1/2 glass bitter gourd juice
- 7-8 fresh great basil leaves

Preparation: Mix honey with crushed basil leaves and bitter gourd juice.

How to take it: In the morning, 30 minutes before meal.

Tips:

- Bitter gourd properties: contains vitamins (A, B complex, C, E, K) and minerals (calcium, magnesium, iron, manganese, zinc, phosphorous), polypeptide-P, charantin, flavonoids (alpha- and beta-carotene, lutein, zeaxanthin), high amount of fibers; antibiotic, anti-oxidant, anti-inflammatory, anti-parasitic, boosts immune system, helps with cough, lowers blood sugar, lowers cholesterol, laxative, anti-cancer.
- Bitter gourd beneficial effects: respiratory infections, asthma, urinary infections, high blood

pressure, rheumatism, psoriasis, Type 2 diabetes, constipation.
- Great basil properties: contains vitamins (A, B complex, C, E, K), minerals (calcium, magnesium, potassium, phosphorous, manganese, zinc, iron), flavonoids (lutein, zeaxanthin, vicenin, orientin, beta-carotene), essential oils (eugenol, cineole, citronelol, estragole, limonene, sabinene, linalool, myrcene); anti-oxidant, strong anti-inflammatory, reduces fever, stimulates appetite, reduces flatulence, lowers cholesterol.
- Great basil beneficial effects: respiratory and urinary infections, asthma, arthritis, dyspepsia, flatulence, irritable bowel, cardio-vascular diseases, skin infections, kidney stones, menstrual pain, headaches.
- Use organic raw honey, bitter gourd and basil.
- Use regularly for better effects

Precautions:

- Bitter gourd contraindications: pregnancy, persons with hypoglycemia.
- Great basil contraindications: pregnancy.
- Do not use if you are allergic to any ingredient
- Contact your doctor with any questions or concerns

Disclaimer: This does not replace medical advice. Check With Your Doctor for symptoms or worsening of condition.

Chapter 5

Cardio-vascular Diseases

Arterial Hypertension (High Blood Pressure)

Arterial hypertension is a chronic condition in which there are repeated high blood pressure values, either only of the systolic pressure (the first measured value), or of both the systolic and the diastolic pressure (both measured values).

Symptoms (rare):

- headaches
- tinnitus (buzzing in the ears)
- lightheadedness

Complications:

High blood pressure leads to pathologic changes in the blood vessels, thus damaging most organs. Heart, brain and kidneys are especially affected.

- stroke
- coronary artery disease, myocardial infarction (heart attack)
- chronic kidney disease
- retinopathy
- peripheral vascular disease etc.

Risk Factors:

- cholesterol: high LDL and low HDL cholesterol
- smoking
- obesity
- sedentary lifestyle
- diabetes

Recipe 20 - Honey and Cucumber

Difficulty: +; Time: 15 minutes;

Ingredients:

- 1 1/2 tablespoon honey
- 3 medium cucumbers

Preparation: Mix honey with blended cucumbers. Store in the fridge.

How to take it: 1/3 of the mixture, 3 times a day, 30 minutes before meals.

Tips:

- Cucumber properties: 95% water, vitamins (A, B complex, C, K), minerals (calcium, magnesium, potassium, iron, phosphorous, molybdenum, selenium, zinc), flavonoids (quercetin, apigenin, kaempherol, alpha- and beta-caroten, lutein, zeaxanthin), triterpenes (cucurbitacin A, B, C, D), lignans (lariciresinol, pinoresinol); stimulates blood circulation, anti-oxidant, anti-inflammatory, hydrating, diuretic, astringent, dissolves uric acid and urates.

- Cucumber beneficial effects: high blood pressure, gout, arthritis, kidney stones, constipation, helps with weight-loss, detoxification. Skin benefits in acne, dermatitis, sunburns.
- Use organic raw honey and cucumbers.
- Use in 1 week cure every 2-3 months for better effects

Precautions:

- Cucumber contraindications: severe high blood pressure, ascitis, and other conditions with fluid retention.
- Do not use if you are allergic to any ingredient
- Contact your doctor with any questions or concerns

Disclaimer: This does not replace medical advice. Check With Your Doctor for symptoms or worsening of condition.

Recipe 21 - Honey and Dill Seeds

Difficulty: +; Time: 15 minutes;

Ingredients:

- 10 tablespoons honey
- 4 tablespoons dill seeds

Preparation: Ground dill seeds in the coffee grinder, then mix with honey. Store in the fridge.

How to take it: 1 tablespoon mixed in 1 glass of water, in the morning, 30 minutes before meal.

Tips:

- Dill properties: contains vitamins (A, B complex, C), minerals (potassium, calcium, magnesium, phosphorous, manganese), flavonoids (beta-carotene equivalents); anti-inflammatory, diuretic, antispastic, lowers cholesterol, estrogenic, stimulates and balances the female hormonal activity, triggers menstruation, stimulates lactate production.
- Dill beneficial effects: high blood pressure, adjuvant in amenorrhea, reduced milk secretion, dysmenorrhea (irregular and painful mentruation), female sterility, premature menopause,

mammary hypoplasia (small breasts), dyspepsia, flatulence (fermentation colitis), gall bladder dyskinesia, urinary infections, helps with weight-loss.
- Use organic raw honey and dill seeds.
- Use regularly for better effects

Precautions:

- Dill contraindications: pregnancy, hyperestrogenism, hypermenorrhea, ovarian cysts, mammary nodules, mammary and genital tumors.
- Do not use if you are allergic to any ingredient
- Contact your doctor with any questions or concerns

Disclaimer: This does not replace medical advice. Check With Your Doctor for symptoms or worsening of condition.

Recipe 22 - Honey and Caraway

Difficulty: +; Time: 2-3 minutes;

Ingredients:

- 1 tablespoon honey
- 1 teaspoon caraway seeds (actual fruits)

Preparation: Mix honey with caraway fruits.

How to take it: In the morning and evening, 30 minutes before meals.

Tips:

- Caraway properties: vitamins (A, B complex, C, E), minerals (calcium, magnesium, zinc, iron, copper, manganese), flavonoids (lutein, beta-carotene, cryptoxanthin), volatile oils (carveol, fufurol, carvone, etc.); lowers cholesterol, anti-oxidant, anti-inflammatory, antiseptic, helps with cough, anti-flatulent, boosts immunity, stimulates and balances the female hormonal activity, triggers menstruation, diminishes pre-menstrual syndrome, stimulates lactate production, vermifuge.
- Caraway beneficial effects: high blood pressure, respiratory and other infections, arthritis,

rheumatism, gout, dyspepsia, irritable bowel syndrome, antihelmintic (intestinal worms), reduced milk secretion, pre-menstrual syndrome, dysmenorrhea (irregular and painful mentruation).

- Use organic raw honey and caraway.
- Use regularly for better effects

Precautions:

- Caraway seeds contraindications: high doses may affect kidneys and liver.
- Do not use if you are allergic to any ingredient
- Contact your doctor with any questions or concerns

Disclaimer: This does not replace medical advice. Check With Your Doctor for symptoms or worsening of condition.

Recipe 23 - Honey and Great Basil

Difficulty: +; Time: 3 minutes;

Ingredients:

- 1 tablespoon honey
- 1 teaspoon chopped fresh basil leaves

Preparation: Mix honey with basil leaves.

How to take it: In the morning, 30 minutes before meal.

Tips:

- Great basil properties: contains vitamins (A, B complex, C, E, K), minerals (calcium, magnesium, potassium, phosphorous, manganese, zinc, iron), flavonoids (lutein, zeaxanthin, vicenin, orientin, beta-carotene), essential oils (eugenol, cineole, citronelol, estragole, limonene, sabinene, linalool, myrcene); anti-oxidant; strong anti-inflammatory; reduces fever; stimulates appetite; reduces flatulence; lowers cholesterol.
- Great basil beneficial effects: respiratory and urinary infections, asthma, arthritis, dyspep-

sia, flatulence, irritable bowel, cardio-vascular diseases, skin infections, kidney stones, menstrual pain, headaches.

- Use organic raw honey and basil
- Use regularly for better effects

Precautions:

- Great basil contraindications: pregnancy.
- Do not use if you are allergic to any ingredient
- Contact your doctor with any questions or concerns

Disclaimer: This does not replace medical advice. Check With Your Doctor for symptoms or worsening of condition.

Recipe 24 - Honey and Garlic

Difficulty: +; Time: 5-minute preparation; 3-day maceration;

Ingredients:

- 9 tablespoons honey
- 10 garlic cloves

Preparation: Mix honey with crushed cloves to make a paste. Store in the fridge for 3 days.

How to take it: 1 tablespoon 30 minutes before meals, in the morning and in the evening.

Tips:

- Garlic properties: contains vitamins (A, B complex, C, K), minerals (calcium, magnesium, iron, manganese, potassium, selenium, zinc, phosphorous), thiosulfinates (allicin, methyl allyl sulfinates), ajoenes, sulfides, sulfoxides (alliin, isoalliin, methiin, garlicins), flavonoids (beta-carotene, lutein, zeaxanthin); anti-bacterial, anti-viral, anti-fungal, anti-inflammatory, anti-oxidant, anti-platelet activity, decreases cholesterol, lowers blood sugar, lowers blood pressure.

- Garlic beneficial effects: heart diseases, high blood pressure, various cancers, respiratory infections, sinusitis, asthma, gastric and duodenal ulcers, especially associated with *Helicobacter pylori*, liver cirrhosis, osteoporosis, improves performance and reduces fatigue, detoxifies the body of heavy metals.
- Use organic raw honey and garlic.
- Use regularly for better effects

Precautions:

- Garlic: may lower Saquinavir levels and may interact with some anticoagulants and diabetes medication. If you are on anticoagulants (blood thinners), ask your doctor before starting a cure!!! May cause flatulence and nausea. Locally applied may lead to irritation, urticaria, anaphylaxis.
- Do not use if you are allergic to any ingredient
- Contact your doctor with any questions or concerns

Disclaimer: This does not replace medical advice. Check With Your Doctor for symptoms or worsening of condition.

Recipe 25 - Honey, Walnuts and Elderberry Flowers

Difficulty: ++; Time: 45 minutes;

Ingredients:

- 150 g honey
- 1 teaspoon elderberry flowers
- 100 g walnuts

Preparation: Grind the walnuts, and mix with the elderberry flowers. Add 500 ml water and boil for 30 minutes in small heat. Let it cool, filter, then mix with honey. Store in the fridge.

How to take it: 1 tablespoon, 30 minutes before meals, 3 times a day.

Tips:

- Walnuts properties: vitamins (A, B complex, E), minerals (magnesium, zinc, manganese, molybdenum, copper, iron), flavonoids (beta-carotene, lutein, zeaxanthin), proteins (contain L-arginine, which is an essential amino acid); anti-oxidant, anti-inflammatory, lower cholesterol, increase insulin production, laxative.

- Walnuts beneficial effects: prevention of cardio-vascular diseases; lower blood pressure; prevent macular degeneration and cataract, asthma, rheumatoid arthritis, psoriasis, eczema; improve depression; prevent gallstones, constipation, Type 2 diabetes; great for hair and skin.
- Elderberry flowers properties: vitamins (A, B complex, C), minerals (calcium, potassium, phosphorous, iron, manganese), tannins, sterols, sugars (among which cyanogenic glycosides), flavonoids (quercetin, beta-carotene), fatty acids; anti-oxidant; lower cholesterol, anti-inflammatory; expectorant; astringent; boost immunity; diuretic; mild laxative.
- Elderberry flowers beneficial effects: lower blood pressure, respiratory infections, asthma, sinusitis, sore throat, ear infections, skin infections (acne, boils, skin rashes), rheumatism, arthritis, gout; help with kidney stones, constipation.
- Use organic raw honey, walnuts and elderberry flowers.
- Following the cure, repeat it after 1 month

Precautions:

- Walnuts: may trigger allergy, even anaphylaxis; when used on skin may cause rash; may cause loose stools.
- Elderberry: contraindications in acute and chronic diarrhea. In high doses (over 200 g per day), may lead to intoxication (throat irritation, heartburn, nausea and vomiting, trouble breathing, convulsions).

- Do not use if you are allergic to any ingredient
- Contact your doctor with any questions or concerns

Disclaimer: This does not replace medical advice. Check With Your Doctor for symptoms or worsening of condition.

Recipe 26 - Honey, Red Beets, Lemon and Carrot

Difficulty: +; Time: 5 minutes;

Ingredients:

- 300 g honey
- 250 ml red beet juice
- juice from 1 lemon
- 250 ml carrot juice

Preparation: Mix honey with red beat, lemon and carrot juices. Store in the fridge.

How to take it: 1 tablespoon 30 minutes before meals, 3 times a day.

Tips:

- Red beets properties: contain vitamins (A, B complex, C, E, K), minerals (calcium, magnesium, copper, manganese), flavonoids (high content beta-caroten, lutein), high content in carbohydrates, betalains (vulgaxanthin, betanin); anti-oxidant, anti-inflammatory, detoxifying, lower cholesterol.
- Red beets beneficial effects: anemia, help prevent macular degeneration and cataracts, skin conditions, constipation.

- Carrot properties: contains vitamins (A, B complex, C, E, K), minerals (copper, manganese, molybdenum), carotenoids (alfa- and beta-caroten, lutein), anthocyanindins, hydroxycinamic acid, high fiber content; anti-oxidant, anti-inflammatory, antibacterial, detoxifying, lowers cholesterol, lowers insulin resistance, boosts immunity.
- Carrot beneficial effects: prevents macular degeneration, improves vision, prevents heart disease, stroke, helps with gum and teeth disorders, improves digestion, anti-cancer.
- Lemon properties: contains vitamins (A, B complex, C, E), minerals (calcium, magnesium, potassium, copper, manganese, zinc, iron), flavonoids (naringin, naringenin, hesperetin, alfa- and beta-carotenes, lutein, zeaxanthin, beta-cryptoxanthin, tannins), terpenes, citric acid, fibers; anti-oxidant, anti-inflammatory, anti-bacterial, antifungal, antiseptic, immune system booster.
- Lemon beneficial effects: dyspepsia, constipation, respiratory infections, asthma, rheumatism, arthritis, lowers blood pressure, helps with weight-loss, anti-cancer, acne, eczema, burns.
- Use organic raw honey, red beets, carrots and lemon.

Precautions:

- Red beets may cause rarely red or pink-colored urine (beeturia), especially in people with iron deficiency; less commonly, color the stools in red. Avoid eating in excess - may induce kidney or gall-bladder stones.

- Consumed in excess, carrots may color the skin orange (face, palms, feet). Avoid in small intestine inflammation, acute gastro-duodenal ulcer.
- Lemon may cause photosensitivity when used on skin.
- Do not use if you are allergic to any ingredient
- Contact your doctor with any questions or concerns

Disclaimer: This does not replace medical advice. Check With Your Doctor for symptoms or worsening of condition.

Coronary Artery Disease (Ischemic Heart Disease)

CAD represents a group of cardiovascular diseases, where the blood supply to the heart is limited, because of narrowed and hardened coronary arteries (the heart's arteries), following plaque development on their inner walls. The process is called atherosclerosis, and the plaque consists of cholesterol, other fats, living and dead blood cells, as well as crystals of calcium and other materials.

The diseases included in this group are the stable and unstable anginas, the myocardial infarction (heart attack) and sudden cardiac death.

Symptoms:

- chest pain (angina) - the cardinal symptom, usually occurs during physical effort or because of stress, but also at rest in case of advanced disease
- shortness of breath
- palpitations
- nausea
- dizziness

Risk Factors:

- cholesterol: high LDL and low HDL cholesterol
- smoking
- obesity
- sedentary lifestyle
- high blood pressure
- diabetes

Recipe 27 - Honey, Corn Oil and Egg White

Difficulty: +; Time: 15 minutes;

Ingredients:

- 400 g honey
- 10 ml corn oil
- 4 egg whites

Preparation: Mix honey with corn oil and whipped egg whites. Store in the fridge.

How to take it: 1 tablespoon in the morning, 30 minutes before meal.

Tips:

- Corn oil properties: contains vitamins (B complex, C, D, E, K), choline, mono- and polyunsaturated fats, essential fatty acids (omega 3 and 6), minerals (iron, copper, aluminum, manganese, chromium), phytosterols; lowers cholesterol, boosts immune system, anti-oxidant.
- Corn oil beneficial effects: helps in coronary disease, arteritis, lowers high blood pressure, gout, rheumatism, gastritis.

- Egg white properties: contains vitamins (B complex), minerals (calcium, magnesium, potassium, iron), high amounts of proteins, enzymes.
- Use organic raw honey, eggs and corn oil.

Precautions:

- Do not use if you are allergic to any ingredient
- Contact your doctor with any questions or concerns

Disclaimer: This does not replace medical advice. Check With Your Doctor for symptoms or worsening of condition.

Recipe 28 - Honey and Horseradish

Difficulty: +; Time: 10 minutes;

Ingredients:

- 500 g honey
- 200 g horseradish

Preparation: Mix honey with grated horseradish root to make a paste. Store in the fridge.

How to take it: 1 tablespoon in the morning 30 minutes before meal.

Tips:

- Horseradish properties: contains vitamins (A, B complex, C - high content), minerals (calcium, magnesium, iron, phosphorous, zinc, copper, manganese), flavonoids (beta-carotene, lutein, zeaxanthin) glutamines, asparagine, sinigrin (a glucosinolate), allyl isothiocyanate; cardiotonic, anti-oxidant, anti-inflammatory, relaxant, expectorant, laxative.
- Horseradish beneficial effects: lowers blood pressure, helps in angina pectoris, respiratory infections, cold, sinusitis, bronchitis, asthma, helps in anorexia etc.

- Use organic raw honey and horseradish.
- Use for 30 days. The cure may be repeated after 3 months.

Precautions:

- Horseradish contraindications: palpitations (cardiac rhythm disturbances), hemorrhoids.
- Do not use if you are allergic to any ingredient
- Contact your doctor with any questions or concerns

Disclaimer: This does not replace medical advice. Check With Your Doctor for symptoms or worsening of condition.

Honey and Turmeric - see recipe 6

Recipe 29 - Honey and Common Sea Buckthorn

Difficulty: +; Time: 30 minutes;

Ingredients:

- 6 tablespoons honey
- 2 tablespoons dry sea buckthorn
- 1 l milk

Preparation: Grind the dry sea buckthorn and mix it with hot milk. Let it infuse for 20 minutes, then let it cool and filter it. Mix liquid with honey. Store in the fridge.

How to take it: 150 ml after meal, 3 times a day.

Tips:

- Sea buckthorn properties: contains vitamins (A, B complex, C - high content, E, F, K, P), minerals (magnesium, calcium, phosphorus), flavonoids (quercetin, kaempherol, isorhamnetin, alpha- and beta-carotenoids, lutein, zeaxanthin, lycopene, catechins, epigallocatechins, gallocatechins), phytosterols, omega-3, omega-6, omega-7, omega-9 fatty acids, essential amino acids, tannins etc.; antioxidant, anti-inflammatory, stimulates immunity and wound healing.

- Sea buckthorn beneficial effects: infections (especially respiratory), digestive tract disorders (gastric ulcer, hepatitis), high blood pressure, coronary disease, eye disorders, skin conditions (eczema, psoriasis, dermatitis), rheumatism, neurologic disorders (asthenia, depression, Parkinson, Alzheimer).
- Use organic raw honey and sea buckthorn
- Use regularly for a month. After 1-2 weeks pause, repeat the cure.

Precautions:

- Sea buckthorn contraindications: in inflammation of the gall bladder (acute cholecystitis) and pancreas (pancreatitis). It may lead to mastopathy in women and to adenomatous prostatitis (high content in phytohormones) in men, and, in high amounts, may lead to allergies as well, in asthma and in rarely cases due to high quantities of beta-caroten.
- Do not use if you are allergic to any ingredient
- Contact your doctor with any questions or concerns

Disclaimer: This does not replace medical advice. Check With Your Doctor for symptoms or worsening of condition.

Recipe 30 - Honey, Lemon, Red Onion and Garlic

Difficulty: ++; Time: 30 minutes;

Ingredients:

- 300 g honey
- 2 lemons
- 1 garlic bulb
- 2 red onions
- 1 liter boiled water

Preparation: Mix lemon with red onion and garlic juice. Add boiled water and let it cool. Then mix with honey and store it in the fridge for 2 days.

How to take it: 1 teaspoon before meals, 3 times a day.

Tips:

- Lemon properties: contains vitamins (A, B complex, C, E), minerals (calcium, magnesium, potassium, copper, manganese, zinc, iron), flavonoids (naringin, naringenin, hesperetin, alfa- and beta-carotenes, lutein, zeaxanthin, beta-cryptoxanthin, tannins), terpenes, citric acid, fibers; anti-oxidant, anti-inflammatory, anti-bacterial, antifungal, antiseptic, immune system booster.

- Lemon beneficial effects: dyspepsia, constipation, respiratory infections, asthma, rheumatism, arthritis, lowers blood pressure, helps with weight-loss, anti-cancer, acne, eczema, burns.
- Onion properties: contains vitamins (B complex, C, D), minerals (calcium, magnesium, potassium, copper, phosphorus, manganese), flavonoids (quercetin, fisetin, tannins, anthocyanins), thiosulfinates, fiber; anti-oxidant, anti-inflammatory, decreases cholesterol, improves mood and lowers blood sugar, anti-cancer.
- Onion beneficial effects: prevention and improvement in heart diseases, respiratory infections, asthma, sinusitis, depression, improves sleep.
- Garlic properties: contains vitamins (A, B complex, C, K), minerals (calcium, magnesium, iron, manganese, potassium, selenium, zinc, phosphorous), thiosulfinates (allicin, methyl allyl sulfinates), ajoenes, sulfides, sulfoxides (alliin, isoalliin, methiin, garlicins), flavonoids (beta-carotene, lutein, zeaxanthin); anti-bacterial, anti-viral, anti-fungal, anti-inflammatory, anti-oxidant, anti-platelet activity, decreases cholesterol, lowers blood sugar, lowers blood pressure.
- Garlic beneficial effects: heart diseases, high blood pressure, various cancers, respiratory infections, sinusitis, asthma, gastric and duodenal ulcers, especially associated with *Helicobacter pylori*, liver cirrhosis, osteoporosis, improves performance and reduces fatigue, detoxifies the body of heavy metals.

- Use organic raw honey, lemon, red onions and garlic.
- Use regularly for better effects

Precautions:

- Lemon may cause photosensitivity when used on skin.
- Red onion may cause bloating, in high amounts may interfere with blood thinning. If you are on anticoagulants (blood thinners), ask your doctor before starting a cure!!!
- Garlic: may lower Saquinavir levels and may interact with some anticoagulants and diabetes medication. If you are on anticoagulants (blood thinners), ask your doctor before starting a cure!!! May cause flatulence and nausea. Locally applied may lead to irritation, urticaria, anaphylaxis.
- Do not use if you are allergic to any ingredient
- Contact your doctor with any questions or concerns

Disclaimer: This does not replace medical advice. Check With Your Doctor for symptoms or worsening of condition.

Recipe 31 - Honey, Lemon and Garlic

Difficulty: ++; Time: 15 minutes; 1 week to macerate;

Ingredients:
- 500 g honey
- 5 lemons
- 3 bulbs garlic

Preparation: Crush the garlic, then mix it with honey and lemon juice. Let it macerate in the fridge for 1 week.

How to take it: 2-3 teaspoons 30 minutes before meals in the morning or evening.

Tips:
- Lemon properties: contains vitamins (A, B complex, C, E), minerals (calcium, magnesium, potassium, copper, manganese, zinc, iron), flavonoids (naringin, naringenin, hesperetin, alfa- and beta-carotenes, lutein, zeaxanthin, beta-cryptoxanthin, tannins), terpenes, citric acid, fibers; anti-oxidant, anti-inflammatory, anti-bacterial, antifungal, antiseptic, immune system booster.

- Lemon beneficial effects: dyspepsia, constipation, respiratory infections, asthma, rheumatism, arthritis, lowers blood pressure, helps with weight-loss, anti-cancer, acne, eczema, burns.
- Garlic properties: contains vitamins (A, B complex, C, K), minerals (calcium, magnesium, iron, manganese, potassium, selenium, zinc, phosphorous), thiosulfinates (allicin, methyl allyl sulfinates), ajoenes, sulfides, sulfoxides (alliin, isoalliin, methiin, garlicins), flavonoids (beta-carotene, lutein, zeaxanthin); anti-bacterial, anti-viral, anti-fungal, anti-inflammatory, anti-oxidant, anti-platelet activity, decreases cholesterol, lowers blood sugar, lowers blood pressure.
- Garlic beneficial effects: heart diseases, high blood pressure, various cancers, respiratory infections, sinusitis, asthma, gastric and duodenal ulcers, especially associated with *Helicobacter pylori*, liver cirrhosis, osteoporosis, improves performance and reduces fatigue, detoxifies the body of heavy metals.
- Use organic raw honey, lemon and garlic.
- Use regularly for better effects

Precautions:

- Lemon may cause photosensitivity when used on skin.
- Garlic: may lower Saquinavir levels and may interact with some anticoagulants and diabetes medication. If you are on anticoagulants (blood thinners), ask your doctor before starting a cure!!!

May cause flatulence and nausea. Locally applied may lead to irritation, urticaria, anaphylaxis.
- Do not use if you are allergic to any ingredient
- Contact your doctor with any questions or concerns

Disclaimer: This does not replace medical advice. Check With Your Doctor for symptoms or worsening of condition.

Cardiac Insufficiency (Heart Failure)

Heart failure develop when the heart is no more able to properly pump blood, so that the body's needs are no more met.

Symptoms:

- shortness of breath (dyspnoea) by physical effort or even at rest
- palpitations
- repeated cough, with white or sometimes blood-tinged flegma
- leg swelling (edema), in advanced cases even ascites
- fatigability and weakness
- increased urination at night

Risk Factors:

- other cardiovascular conditions, such as: coronary artery disease, heart attack, high blood pressure, congenital heart diseases, rhythm disturbances (palpitations) and others
- diabetes and in some persons oral hypoglycemics such as rosiglitazone and pioglitazone

- alcohol use
- tobacco use
- obesity

Recipe 32 - Honey and Cheese

Difficulty: +; Time: 2-3 minutes;

Ingredients:

- 1 teaspoon honey
- 1 teaspoon cottage cheese

Preparation: Mix honey with cheese.

How to take it: 2-3 times a day, before meals.

Tips:

- Use organic raw honey and cheese.
- Use regularly for better effects

Precautions:

- Do not use if you are allergic to any ingredient
- Contact your doctor with any questions or concerns

Disclaimer: This does not replace medical advice. Check With Your Doctor for symptoms or worsening of condition.

Recipe 33 - Honey and Oats

Difficulty: +; Time: 10 minutes; 24 hours to macerate;

Ingredients:
- 5 tablespoons honey
- 100 g oats
- 1 liter water

Preparation: Mix oats with water and let it macerate for 24 hours. Filter it, then mix it with honey.

How to take it: 1/4 glass 2-3 times a day, 30 minutes before meals.

Tips:
- Oats properties: contain vitamins (A, B complex, C, D, E, F, K), minerals (molybdenum, manganese, magnesium, calcium, phosphorus, selenium, iron, zinc), flavonoids (alfa- and beta-carotenoids), amino acids etc.; anti-oxidant, improve sugar control, have high fiber content and lower cholesterol, expectorant, diuretic.
- Oats beneficial effects: in high blood pressure, in respiratory diseases, in diabetes, help weight loss, in skin conditions (eczema, psoriasis,

urticaria, dermatitis), rheumatism, gout, constipation.
- Use organic raw honey and oats.
- Use regularly for better effects

Precautions:

- Do not use if you are allergic to any ingredient (in oats' case, if gluten or celiac allergy)
- Contact your doctor with any questions or concerns

Disclaimer: This does not replace medical advice. Check With Your Doctor for symptoms or worsening of condition.

Cardiomyopathy

Cardiomyopathy represents a group of diseases in which the heart muscle is altered (thick, enlarged, stiffed, or rarely, scar tissue replaces the muscle).

Symptoms:

- no symptoms in the early stages of disease, and some people may remain asymptomatic
- shortness of breath, especially by physical effort
- swelling of the lower limbs, later of the abdomen
- fatigue
- dizziness
- palpitations

Risk factors:

- alcoholism
- chronic high blood pressure
- other cardiovascular diseases (viral infection of the heart muscle, coronary heart disease,

heart attack) or conditions damaging the heart (amyloidosis, hemochromatosis or sarcoidosis)
- metabolic diseases, such as diabetes or obesity

Recipe 34 - Honey and Common St John's Wort

Difficulty: ++; Time: 30 minutes;

Ingredients:

- 200 g honey
- 50 g St John's Wort
- 1 l water

Preparation: Boil the dried plants in water. Reduce heat and let it simmer for 10-15 minutes. Let it cool and then mix with honey. Store in the fridge.

How to take it: 1/2 glass twice a day, before meals.

Tips:

- Common St John's wort properties: contains vitamins (A, C), flavonoids (beta-caroten, rutin, tannins), dianthrone derivatives (hypericin, pseudohypericin), organic acids, pectin, essential oils (monoterpenes), rezins, coline, coumarins (scopoletine); diuretic, antioxidant and anti-inflammatory, astringent, wound healing, antidepressive, stimulates digestion, fights against diarrhea.
- Common St John's wort beneficial effects: lowers blood pressure, improves digestion, hemorrhoids, anxiety and depression, reduces chronic

fatigue and insomnia, skin wounds (bruises, burns, insect bites and scabies).
- Use organic raw honey and common St John's wort.
- At least 10 days pause between cures.

Precautions:

- Common St John's wort side-effects: dizziness and confusion, gastro-intestinal symptoms (dry mouth, constipation, etc.).
- Common St John's wort contraindications: increases blood pressure through blood vessels narrowing, decreases potency in prolonged use, may cause photo dermatitis. Should not be used with ethinyl estradiol, non-nucleoside reverse transcriptase inhibitors and protease inhibitors in HIV treatment, irinotecan, cyclosporine, imatinib mesylate, tacrolimus.
- Do not use if you are allergic to any ingredient
- Contact your doctor with any questions or concerns

Disclaimer: This does not replace medical advice. Check With Your Doctor for symptoms or worsening of condition.

Varicose veins (varicosities)

Varicose veins is a condition in which the veins are contorted and enlarged. It usually affects lower limbs' veins, however any vein in the body may be affected.

Symptoms:

- pain (achiness, heaviness, burning, itching, throbbing) around the crooked, highly visible veins
- swelling
- discoloration, or even color change with hardening of the vein: this represents a serious condition - seek medical advice!!!
- bleeding

Risk factors:

- sex and age
- prolonged standing or sitting
- obesity
- relatives having varicose veins

Recipe 35 - Honey and Garlic

Difficulty: +; Time: 15 minutes; macerate for 7 days;

Ingredients:

- 500 g honey
- 250 g garlic

Preparation: Mix honey with crushed garlic and let to macerate for 7 days. Store in the fridge.

How to take it: 1 tablespoon 3 times a day, 30 minutes before meals.

Tips:

- Garlic properties: contains vitamins (A, B complex, C, K), minerals (calcium, magnesium, iron, manganese, potassium, selenium, zinc, phosphorous), thiosulfinates (allicin, methyl allyl sulfinates), ajoenes, sulfides, sulfoxides (alliin, isoalliin, methiin, garlicins), flavonoids (beta-carotene, lutein, zeaxanthin); anti-bacterial, anti-viral, anti-fungal, anti-inflammatory, anti-oxidant, anti-platelet activity, decreases cholesterol, lowers blood sugar, lowers blood pressure.

- Garlic beneficial effects: heart diseases, high blood pressure, various cancers, respiratory infections, sinusitis, asthma, gastric and duodenal ulcers, especially associated with *Helicobacter pylori*, liver cirrhosis, osteoporosis, improves performance and reduces fatigue, detoxifies the body of heavy metals.
- Use organic raw honey and garlic.
- Use regularly for better effects

Precautions:

- Garlic: may lower Saquinavir levels and may interact with some anticoagulants and diabetes medication. If you are on anticoagulants (blood thinners), ask your doctor before starting a cure!!! May cause flatulence and nausea. Locally applied may lead to irritation, urticaria, anaphylaxis.
- Do not use if you are allergic to any ingredient
- Contact your doctor with any questions or concerns

Disclaimer: This does not replace medical advice. Check With Your Doctor for symptoms or worsening of condition.

Recipe 36 - Honey and Apple Cider Vinegar

Difficulty: +; Time: 5 minutes;

Ingredients:
- 1 1/2 tablespoon honey
- 1 tablespoon apple cider vinegar
- 1 glass water

Preparation: Mix honey with apple cider vinegar and water, just before taking it.

How to take it: In the morning, 30 minutes before meal and at bed time.

Tips:
- Apple cider vinegar properties: contains vitamins (B complex, C, pantothenic acid), minerals (calcium, potassium, sodium, iron, phosphorus), acetic acid, malic acid, pectin, polyphenols (flavonols, flavanols, tannins, anthocyanins, dihydrochalcones, hydroxycinnamic acids); boosts immunity, anti-microbial, anti-inflammatory, anti-oxidant, lowers cholesterol, lowers blood sugar, acts as anti-acid.

- Apple cider vinegar beneficial effects: in infections (sinusitis, sore throat, asthma, other respiratory infections, urinary tract infections, etc), allergies, arthritis, gout, cardiovascular diseases, improves digestion, prevents constipation, helps with weight loss, in skin conditions (acne, eczema).
- Use organic raw honey and apple cider vinegar.
- Use regularly for 1 month for better effects.

Precautions:

- Do not use if you are allergic to any ingredient
- Contact your doctor with any questions or concerns

Disclaimer: This does not replace medical advice. Check With Your Doctor for symptoms or worsening of condition.

Recipe 37 - Honey and Red Onion Juice

Difficulty: ++; Time: 15 minutes;

Ingredients:

- 250 g honey (preferably Acacia honey)
- 700 ml red onion juice

Preparation: Squeeze the red onions and filter the resulted juice, then mix it with honey. Store in the fridge.

How to take it: 2 tablespoons, 3 times a day, 30 minutes before meals.

Tips:

- Onion properties: contains vitamins (B complex, C, D), minerals (calcium, magnesium, potassium, copper, phosphorus, manganese), flavonoids (quercetin, fisetin, tannins, anthocyanins), thiosulfinates, fiber; anti-oxidant, anti-inflammatory, decreases cholesterol, improves mood and lowers blood sugar, anti-cancer.
- Onion beneficial effects: prevention and improvement in heart diseases, respiratory infections, asthma, sinusitis, depression, improves sleep.

- Use organic raw honey and onion.
- Use regularly 1 month for better effects. After a 1-month pause may be repeated.

Precautions:

- Red onion may cause bloating; in high quantity, may interfere with blood thinning. If you are on anticoagulants (blood thinners), ask your doctor before starting a cure!!!
- Contraindications: gastritis, gastric or duodenal ulcers.
- Do not use if you are allergic to any ingredient
- Contact your doctor with any questions or concerns

Disclaimer: This does not replace medical advice. Check With Your Doctor for symptoms or worsening of condition.

Peripheral artery disease

Peripheral artery disease is characterized by narrowed arteries, and, consequently, a reduced blood flow towards the territories supplied by these arteries. Most commonly, this narrowing takes place in the lower limbs.

Symptoms:

- "crampy" pain (intermittent claudication) - calf, thigh, or hip pain, which persists after discontinuing exercising
- leg numbness, weakness or coldness
- change in the color and poor hair and nail growth
- slow healing wounds on the toes, feet or legs

Risk factors:

- smoking
- obesity
- high cholesterol
- high blood pressure
- diabetes
- relatives with this condition or other cardiovascular diseases

Recipe 38 - Honey and European Mistletoe

Difficulty: +; Time: 5 minutes; macerate for 8 hours (prepare the evening before);

Ingredients:

- 2 tablespoons honey
- 1 1/2 tablespoon dried mistletoe leaves
- 1/2 l water

Preparation: Mix dried mistletoe leaves with water and let it macerate for 8 hours. Then filter it and mix it with honey.

How to take it: 1/3 of the amount, 3 times a day, 30 minutes before meals.

Tips:

- European mistletoe properties: mistletoe contains alkaloids, lectins I, II and III (glycoproteins), arabinogalactan, galacturonan (polysaccharides), viscotoxin (protein), free amino acids, colins, inosytol, and minerals; vasodilator, lowers blood pressure and reduces cardiac rhythm, cardiotonic, haemostatic, anticonvulsive, helps with cough, analgesic.

- European mistletoe beneficial effects: high blood pressure, coronary disease, stroke, tumors, asthma, bronchitis, neuralgia, convulsions, bleeding, sciatic, rheumatic and gout pains.
- Use organic raw honey and mistletoe.

Precautions:

- European mistletoe contraindications: avoid use during pregnancy or lactation. Do not overdose! Higher doses cause intoxication: low pulse, cardiac arrhythmia, even myocardial lesions.
- Do not use if you are allergic to any ingredient
- Contact your doctor with any questions or concerns

Disclaimer: This does not replace medical advice. Check With Your Doctor for symptoms or worsening of condition.

Recipe 39 - Honey and Dog Rose

Difficulty: +; Time: 30 minutes;

Ingredients:

- 1 table spoon honey
- 1 teaspoon dried dog rose fruits
- 250 ml water

Preparation: Put 1 teaspoon dried dog rose in 250 ml boiling water, let it infuse and cool. Mix with honey.

How to take it: 3 times a day, before meals.

Tips:

- Dog rose properties: contains vitamins (A, B complex, C - high amounts, E, F), minerals (magnesium, calcium, manganese, selenium, iron, zinc, phosphorous, sulfur), flavonoids (carotenoids, tannins), terpenoids, organic acids; reduces small blood vessels fragility, anti-oxidant, anti-inflammatory, lowers blood sugar, boosts immunity, promotes regeneration, diuretic, stimulates uric acid removal.

- Dog rose beneficial effects: improves peripheral circulation, reduces atherosclerosis, respiratory and urinary infections, rheumatism, gout, gall bladder disorders, kidney diseases, general tonic.
- Use organic raw honey and dog rose.

Precautions:

- Dog rose contraindications: avoid use during pregnancy or lactation.
- Do not use if you are allergic to any ingredient
- Contact your doctor with any questions or concerns

Disclaimer: This does not replace medical advice. Check With Your Doctor for symptoms or worsening of condition.

Recipe 40 - Honey and Fresh Beer Yeast

Difficulty: +; Time: 5 minutes;

Ingredients:
- 2 tablespoons honey
- 3 teaspoons fresh beer yeast

Preparation: Mix honey with yeast to make a paste. Store in the fridge. Prepare it every day.

How to take it: 3 times a day, 1 hour before meals.

Tips:
- Beer yeast properties: contains vitamins (B complex), minerals (potassium, magnesium, selenium, zinc, copper, iron), beta-1,3 glucan, glutathione, mannan, trehalose; improves blood circulation, balances blood pressure and cholesterol, boosts immunity, anti-aging, helps with calcium storage, prevents constipation, helps with weight-loss, tonic, enhances concentration, decreases fatigue.
- Beer yeast beneficial effects: cardio-vascular diseases, peripheral artheriopathy, metabolic regulation, psoriasis, acne, seborrhea, alopecia, stomatitis, infections, neuro-psychiatric disorders

(Alzheimer, Parkinson, dementia), osteoporosis, andropause, and menopause.
- Use organic raw honey and beer yeast.
- Use for 10-30 days, pause for 1 week, then may repeat.

Precautions:

- Do not use if you are allergic to any ingredient
- Contact your doctor with any questions or concerns

Disclaimer: This does not replace medical advice. Check With Your Doctor for symptoms or worsening of condition.

Recipe 41 - Honey and Dried Beer Yeast

Difficulty: +; Time: 5 minutes;

Ingredients:

- 2 tablespoons honey
- 2 teaspoons dried beer yeast
- 500 ml fresh apple juice

Preparation: Mix honey with yeast and apple juice. Store in the fridge. Prepare it every day.

How to take it: 1/3 of the beverage, 3 times a day, 1 hour before meals.

Tips:

- Beer yeast properties: contains vitamins (B complex), minerals (potassium, magnesium, selenium, zinc, copper, iron), beta-1,3 glucan, glutathione, mannan, trehalose; improves blood circulation, balances blood pressure and cholesterol, boosts immunity, anti-aging, helps with calcium storage, prevents constipation, helps with weight-loss, tonic, enhances concentration, decreases fatigue.

- Beer yeast beneficial effects: cardio-vascular diseases, peripheral artheriopathy, metabolic regulation, psoriasis, acne, seborrhea, alopecia, stomatitis, infections, neuro-psychiatric disorders (Alzheimer, Parkinson, dementia), osteoporosis, andropause, and menopause.
- Use organic raw honey and beer yeast.
- Use for 10-30 days, pause for 1 week, then may repeat.

Precautions:

- Do not use if you are allergic to any ingredient
- Contact your doctor with any questions or concerns

Disclaimer: This does not replace medical advice. Check With Your Doctor for symptoms or worsening of condition.

Chapter 6

Digestive Diseases

Mouth Ulcers

Mouth ulcer is an injury (sore) which occurs in the mouth, usually as a result of local trauma or infection.

Symptoms:

- discomfort
- pain while eating and drinking, especially spicy or acidic foods and drinks
- fever, enlarged lymph nodes, weakness - in severe cases (associated with infections or other conditions)

Gingivitis

Gingivitis is the inflammation (swelling) of the gums, generally caused by poor oral hygiene.

Symptoms:

- swollen gums
- bright or dark red gums
- tender gums
- easily bleeding gums
- receding gums
- bad breath (halitosis)

Recipe 42 - Honey and Cinnamon

Difficulty: +; Time: 2 - 3 minutes;

Ingredients:

- 1 tablespoon honey
- 1 teaspoon cinnamon
- water or tea

Preparation: Mix thoroughly honey and cinnamon with lukewarm water or tea.

How to take it: In the morning, 30 minutes before meal. Take small sips and keep them in the mouth for a while before swallowing.

Tips:

- Cinnamon properties: contains vitamins (A, B complex, C), minerals (calcium, iron, manganese, phosphorous), essential oils (cinnamaldehyde, cinnamyl alcohol, cinnamyl acetate), flavonoids (alpha- and beta-carotens, lutein, zeaxanthin, cryptoxanthin, lycopene); anti-oxidant, anti-inflammatory, antimicrobial, antifungal, analgesic, anti-spastic, anti-parasites, haemostatic, peripheral vasodilator, lowers cholesterol, reduces stress and fatigue, promotes healing, anti-cancer.

- Cinnamon beneficial effects: infections (respiratory, gynecological: leucorrhea, vaginitis; digestive: gingivitis, mouth ulcers, enterocolitis, amoebiasis), dyspepsia, GERD, gastritis, peptic ulcer, asthenia, depression, Alzheimer, regulates menstruation, eczema, helps with weight-loss.
- Use organic raw honey and cinnamon.
- Use regularly for better effects

Precautions:

- Not to be used in pregnancy and in breast-feeding women
- Do not use if you are allergic to any ingredient
- Contact your doctor with any questions or concerns

Disclaimer: This does not replace medical advice. Check With Your Doctor for symptoms or worsening of condition.

Recipe 43 - Honey and Liquorice

Difficulty: +; Time: 2-3 minutes; 8 hours to macerate;

Ingredients:

- 1 tablespoon honey
- 1/2 teaspoon chopped liquorice root
- 1 glass water

Preparation: Mix liquorice with water and let it macerate for 8 hours. Filter it, then mix with honey.

How to take it: Drink small quantities, over the day. Take small sips and keep them in the mouth for a while before swallowing.

Tips:

- Liquorice properties: contains vitamins (B complex, E), minerals (calcium, magnesium, phosphorous, silicon, iron, zinc, selenium), flavonoids (beta-carotene, quercetin), phenol, glycyrrhizin, thymol, glabridin, phytoestrogens; anti-oxidant, anti-inflammatory, expectorant, growth inhibition of *Helicobacter pylori*, anti-tumor, anti-microbial (also anti-Mycobacterial, antiviral), boosts immunity, lowers cholesterol.

- Liquorice beneficial effects: mouth aphtous ulcers, dyspepsia, gastric and duodenal ulcer associated with *Helicobacter pylori*, liver protection, rheumatism, gout, polyarthritis rheumatoides, menopause, pre-menstrual syndrome, chronic fatigue syndrome, pulmonary infections, pulmonary tuberculosis, acne, shingles, helps in HIV infection, prevention and treatment of cardio-vascular diseases.
- Use organic raw honey and liquorice.

Precautions:

- Liquorice should not be administered during pregnancy, while under digitalis or steroids treatment or in case of renal dysfunction with impaired salt excretion. During the cure, a low salt diet is recommended. May cause body fatigue, kidney disorders, irregular menstruation, may interact with diuretics. Prolonged use may cause the retention of fluid in the body, high blood pressure, low blood potassium levels (hypokalemia), and cataracts.
- Do not use if you are allergic to any ingredient
- Contact your doctor with any questions or concerns

Disclaimer: This does not replace medical advice. Check With Your Doctor for symptoms or worsening of condition.

Recipe 47 - Honey, Liquorice and Chamomile

Gastro-Esophageal Reflux Disease (GERD)

GERD is a chronic disease, where stomach's content flows back into the esophagus (food pipe), irritating and damaging its lining.

Risk factors:

- obesity
- smoking
- pregnancy
- hiatal hernia (bulging of the stomach through the diaphragm)
- diabetes
- connective tissue diseases (scleroderma)
- some drugs: antidepressants, antihistamines, sleeping pills, calcium channel blockers.

Symptoms:

- regurgitation of food or sour liquid in the back of the mouth
- heartburn
- chest pain
- sore throat or/and sensation of a lump in the throat
- dry cough
- problematic swallowing
- vomiting

Recipe 44 - Honey and Chamomile

Difficulty: +; Time: 30 minutes;

Ingredients:

- 2 tablespoons honey
- 5 teaspoons dried chamomile flowers
- 750 ml water

Preparation: Infuse the chamomile in boiling water for 10 minutes. Let it cool, then mix it with honey.

How to take it: 1-3 cups per day, between meals.

Tips:

- Chamomile properties: contains vitamins (B1, C), minerals (calcium, manganese, zinc, iron, copper, phosphorous, silicon), flavonoids (apigenin, luteolin, quercetin, rutin), sesquiterpenes (alpha-bisabolol), terpenoids, coumarins (herniarin, umbelliferone), phenylpropanoids (caffeic acid, chlorogenic acid); anti-inflammatory, antiseptic, anti-allergic, antispasmodic/antidiarrheal, analgesic, helps healing, anti-cancer, anxiolytic.
- Chamomile beneficial effects: helps in GERD, stomachaches, irritable bowel disease,

mouth infections (gingivitis, stomatitis, dental abscesses), sore throat, tonsillitis, leucorrhea, skin disorders (acne, eczema).
- Use organic raw honey and chamomile.
- Use regularly for better effects

Precautions:

- Chamomile: do not use in pregnancy. If you are on anticoagulants (blood thinners), ask your doctor before starting a cure!!!
- Do not use if you are allergic to any ingredient
- Contact your doctor with any questions or concerns

Disclaimer: This does not replace medical advice. Check With Your Doctor for symptoms or worsening of condition.

Recipe 45 - Honey and Cinnamon
Recipe 46 - Honey and Ginger
Recipe 47 - Honey, Liquorice and Chamomile

Gastritis

Gastritis includes a group of diseases in which the major characteristic is the stomach's inner layer inflammation. Depending on the onset and symptomatology, there is an acute and a chronic gastritis.

Symptoms:

- stomach pain (burning or gnawing), which is bettered or worsened with food intake
- nausea and vomiting
- fullness sensation after eating

Risk factors:

- stress
- bacterial infection, especially with *Helicobacter pylori*
- alcohol drinking in excess
- smoking
- regular use or high doses of pain relievers (anti-inflammatory drugs, such as aspirin, diclofenac, ibuprofen etc.)

- other diseases: HIV infection, parasites, Crohn's diseases, vitamin B12 deficiency, autoimmune diseases (type 1 diabetes, Hashimoto's disease etc.)

Recipe 45 - Honey and Cinnamon

Difficulty: ++; Time: 30 minutes;

Ingredients:
- 1 1/2 teaspoon honey
- 1 stick cinnamon
- 1 glass water

Preparation: Put cinnamon in water and boil at small heat for a few minutes. Let it cool and then mix honey.

How to take it: 3 times a day, 30 minutes before meals.

Tips:

- Cinnamon properties: contains vitamins (A, B complex, C), minerals (calcium, iron, manganese, phosphorous), essential oils (cinnamaldehyde, cinnamyl alcohol, cinnamyl acetate), flavonoids (alpha- and beta-carotens, lutein, zeaxanthin, cryptoxanthin, lycopene); anti-oxidant, anti-inflammatory, antimicrobial, antifungal, analgesic, anti-spastic, anti-parasites, haemostatic, peripheral vasodilator, lowers cholesterol, reduces stress and fatigue, promotes healing, anti-cancer.

- Cinnamon beneficial effects: infections (respiratory, gynecological: leucorrhea, vaginitis; digestive: gingivitis, mouth ulcers, enterocolitis, amoebiasis), dyspepsia, GERD, gastritis, peptic ulcer, asthenia, depression, Alzheimer, regulates menstruation, eczema, helps with weight-loss.
- Use organic raw honey and cinnamon.
- Use regularly for better effects

Precautions:
- Do not use if you are allergic to any ingredient
- Contact your doctor with any questions or concerns

Disclaimer: This does not replace medical advice. Check With Your Doctor for symptoms or worsening of condition.

Recipe 44 - Honey and Chamomile

Recipe 46 - Honey and Ginger

Recipe 47 - Honey, Liquorice and Chamomile

Peptic Ulcer Disease (Gastric and Duodenal Ulcer)

Peptic ulcers are lesions (sores) in the inner lining of the stomach and duodenum (rarely in the distal part of the esophagus).

Symptoms:

- stomach pain (burning pain), usually after meal
- heartburn
- fullness sensation and bloating
- intolerance to fats

Severe Symptoms:

- nausea, vomiting, loss of appetite and weight-loss
- hematemesis (blood vomiting) and melena (black stools, which contain digested blood)
- excruciating, stabbing abdominal pain occurs in peptic ulcer perforation, requires emergency surgery!

Risk factors:

- stress
- bacterial infection, especially with *Helicobacter pylori*
- alcohol drinking in excess
- smoking
- spicy foods
- regular use or high doses of pain relievers (anti-inflammatory drugs, such as aspirin, diclofenac, ibuprofen etc.), steroids, alendronate (Fosamax), risedronate (Actonel), serotonergic antidepressants (Citalopram, Escitalopram, Sertraline, Fluvoxamine, Fluoxetine, Paroxetine).

Recipe 46 - Honey and Ginger

Difficulty: ++; Time: 30 minutes;

Ingredients:
- 1 1/2 teaspoon honey
- 1 teaspoon grated ginger
- 1 glass water

Preparation: Put grated ginger in boiling water. Let it cool, filter, then mix with honey.

How to take it: 3 times a day, 30 minutes before meals.

Tips:
- Ginger properties: contains vitamins (B complex, C, E), minerals (calcium, magnesium, phosphorous, potassium, sodium, zinc, iron), gingerols, zingerone, shogaols (volatile oils), beta-carotene, capsaicin, caffeic acid, curcumin, salicylate; anti-oxidant, anti-inflammatory, antibacterial, antifungal, analgesic, anti-nausea, lowers cholesterol, choleretic, anti-cancer.
- Ginger beneficial effects: respiratory infections, asthma, heart disease, GERD, stomach ulcer, diabetes prevention and therapy, weight loss.

- Use organic raw honey and ginger.
- Use regularly for better effects

Precautions:

- Ginger should be avoided in pregnancy and breastfeeding. It may cause blood thinning. If you are on anticoagulants (blood thinners), ask your doctor before starting a cure!!! Precaution is advised when using blood pressure medication.
- Do not use if you are allergic to any ingredient
- Contact your doctor with any questions or concerns

Disclaimer: This does not replace medical advice. Check With Your Doctor for symptoms or worsening of condition.

Recipe 47 - Honey, Liquorice and Chamomile

Difficulty: +; Time: 30 minutes;

Ingredients:

- 2 tablespoons honey
- 1/2 teaspoon chopped liquorice root
- 1 teaspoon chamomile
- 1 glass water

Preparation: Infuse the liquorice and chamomile in boiling water for 10 minutes. Let them cool, then mix them with honey.

How to take it: 1/3 of the amount 3 times a day, 30 minutes before meals.

Tips:

- Liquorice properties: contains vitamins (B complex, E), minerals (calcium, magnesium, phosphorous, silicon, iron, zinc, selenium), flavonoids (beta-carotene, quercetin), phenol, glycyrrhizin, thymol, glabridin, phytoestrogens; anti-oxidant, anti-inflammatory, expectorant, growth inhibition of *Helicobacter pylori,* anti-tumor, anti-microbial (also anti-Mycobacterial, antiviral), boosts immunity, lowers cholesterol.

- Liquorice beneficial effects: mouth aphtous ulcers, dyspepsia, gastric and duodenal ulcer associated with *Helicobacter pylori*, liver protection, rheumatism, gout, polyarthritis rheumatoides, menopause, pre-menstrual syndrome, chronic fatigue syndrome, pulmonary infections, pulmonary tuberculosis, acne, shingles, helps in HIV infection, prevention and treatment of cardio-vascular diseases.
- Chamomile properties: contains vitamins (B1, C), minerals (calcium, manganese, zinc, iron, copper, phosphorous, silicon), flavonoids (apigenin, luteolin, quercetin, rutin), sesquiterpenes (alpha-bisabolol), terpenoids, coumarins (herniarin, umbelliferone), phenylpropanoids (caffeic acid, chlorogenic acid); anti-inflammatory, antiseptic, anti-allergic, antispasmodic/antidiarrheal, analgesic, helps healing, anti-cancer, anxiolytic.
- Chamomile beneficial effects: helps in GERD, stomachaches, irritable bowel disease, mouth infections (gingivitis, stomatitis, dental abscesses), sore throat, tonsillitis, leucorrhea, skin disorders (acne, eczema).
- Use organic raw honey, liquorice and chamomile.
- Use regularly for better effects

Precautions:

- Liquorice should not be administered during pregnancy, while under digitalis or steroids treatment or in case of renal dysfunction with impaired salt excretion. During the cure, a low salt diet is recommended. May cause body fatigue, kidney disorders, irregular menstruation, may interact with diuretics. Prolonged use may cause the retention of fluid in the body, high blood pressure, low blood potassium levels (hypokalemia), and cataracts.

- Chamomile: do not use in pregnancy. If you are on anticoagulants (blood thinners), ask your doctor before starting a cure!!!
- Do not use if you are allergic to any ingredient
- Contact your doctor with any questions or concerns

Disclaimer: This does not replace medical advice. Check With Your Doctor for symptoms or worsening of condition.

Recipe 44 - Honey and Chamomile

Recipe 45 - Honey and Cinnamon

Dyspepsia (Indigestion)

Indigestion is a general term including disturbances in the digestive process. It is most often an expression of another digestive disease (GERD, gastritis, peptic ulcer disease, stomach cancer), or, in about 10 % of cases, there is no organic substrate, the so-called functional dyspepsia.

Symptoms:

- feeling of fullness during a meal or uncomfortable sensation of fullness following a meal
- pain in the stomach area (burning or discomfort)
- bloating
- nausea and vomiting

Seek medical advice when experiencing severe pain, lack of appetite and weight-loss, difficulty swallowing, persistent vomiting or blood in the vomiting, black, tarry stools, fatigue.

Risk factors:

- anxiety and stress
- smoking
- eating fast and overeating
- excessive alcohol, caffeine, carbonated beverages
- spicy and fatty foods
- drugs (certain pain relievers, antibiotics, iron supplements)

Recipe 48 - Honey and Apple Cider Vinegar

Difficulty: +; Time: 2-3 minutes;

Ingredients:

- 1 tablespoon honey
- 3 teaspoons of apple cider vinegar
- 1 glass with water

Preparation: Mix honey with water and apple cider vinegar.

How to take it: Drink it 10 minutes before lunch.

Tips:

- Apple cider vinegar properties: contains vitamins (B complex, C, pantothenic acid), minerals (calcium, potassium, sodium, iron, phosphorus), acetic acid, malic acid, pectin, polyphenols (flavonols, flavanols, tannins, anthocyanins, dihydrochalcones, dydroxycinnamic acids); boosts immunity, anti-microbial, anti-inflammatory, anti-oxidant, lowers cholesterol, lowers blood sugar, acts as anti-acid.
- Apple cider vinegar beneficial effects: in infections (sinusitis, sore throat, asthma, other respiratory infections, urinary tract infections, etc.),

allergies, arthritis, gout, cardiovascular diseases, improves digestion, prevents constipation, helps with weight loss, in skin conditions (acne, eczema).
- Use organic raw honey and apple cider vinegar.
- Use regularly for better effects

Precautions:

- Do not use if you are allergic to any ingredient
- Contact your doctor with any questions or concerns

Disclaimer: This does not replace medical advice. Check With Your Doctor for symptoms or worsening of condition.

Recipe 44 - Honey and Chamomile
Recipe 45 - Honey and Cinnamon
Recipe 47 - Honey, Liquorice and Chamomile

Biliary Lithiasis (Gallstones)

Biliary lithiasis is a condition characterized by the presence of stone(s) in the gall bladder.

Symptoms: in most cases, there are no symptoms.
- crampy pain in the right upper side of the abdomen, may irradiate toward back, between the shoulder blades and in the right shoulder
- nausea, vomiting

Severe symptoms: requires emergency medical treatment!
- yellowing of the whites of the eyes and of the skin (jaundice)
- sudden and extreme pain in the right upper side of the abdomen
- high fever with chills

Risk factors:

- female age 40 or older
- life-style (sedentarism, overweight, high-fat and cholesterol diet, low-fiber diet)
- quick weight-loss, treatment with Orlistat (weight loss drug)
- relatives with gallstones
- drugs containing estrogen (hormone therapy, oral contraceptives), proton pump inhibitors (Omeprazole) used over long periods of time
- diabetes

Recipe 49 - Honey and Liquorice

Difficulty: +; Time: 30 minutes;

Ingredients:

- 4 teaspoons honey
- 2 teaspoons dried liquorice
- 500 ml water

Preparation: Put liquorice in boiling water and let it infuse and cool. Filter it, then mix with honey.

How to take it: Drink 1 cup twice a day, 30 minutes before meals.

Tips:

- Liquorice properties: contains vitamins (B complex, E), minerals (calcium, magnesium, phosphorous, silicon, iron, zinc, selenium), flavonoids (beta-carotene, quercetin), phenol, glycyrrhizin, thymol, glabridin, phytoestrogens; anti-oxidant, anti-inflammatory, expectorant, growth inhibition of *Helicobacter pylori*, anti-tumor, anti-microbial (also anti-Mycobacterial, antiviral), boosts immunity, lowers cholesterol.

- Liquorice beneficial effects: mouth aphtous ulcers, dyspepsia, gastric and duodenal ulcer associated with *Helicobacter pylori*, liver protection, rheumatism, gout, polyarthritis rheumatoides, menopause, pre-menstrual syndrome, chronic fatigue syndrome, pulmonary infections, pulmonary tuberculosis, acne, shingles, helps in HIV infection, prevention and treatment of cardio-vascular diseases.
- Use organic raw honey and liquorice.

Precautions:

- Liquorice should not be administered during pregnancy, while under digitalis or steroids treatment or in case of renal dysfunction with impaired salt excretion. During the cure, a low salt diet is recommended. May cause body fatigue, kidney disorders, irregular menstruation, may interact with diuretics. Prolonged use may cause the retention of fluid in the body, high blood pressure, low blood potassium levels (hypokalemia), and cataracts. Use in 4 to 6-week cure, followed by 2 to 3-week pause.
- Do not use if you are allergic to any ingredient
- Contact your doctor with any questions or concerns

Disclaimer: This does not replace medical advice. Check With Your Doctor for symptoms or worsening of condition.

Recipe 50 - Honey and Dog Rose

Difficulty: ++; Time: 12 hours;

Ingredients:

- 2 tablespoons honey
- 4-5 tablespoons powdered dog rose
- 600 ml water

Preparation: Macerate 4-5 tablespoons powdered dog rose in 300 ml water for 10 hours, then filter it. Boil the filtered plant residue in another 300-ml water for 5 minutes and let it cool. Mix the two solutions, add honey and stir thoroughly. Store in the fridge.

How to take it: 200 ml 3 times a day, 30 minutes before meals.

Tips:

- Dog rose properties: contains vitamins (A, B complex, C - high amounts, E, F), minerals (magnesium, calcium, manganese, selenium, iron, zinc, phosphorous, sulfur), flavonoids (carotenoids, tannins), terpenoids, organic acids; reduces small blood vessels fragility, anti-oxidant, anti-inflam-

matory, lowers blood sugar, boosts immunity, promotes regeneration, diuretic, stimulates uric acid removal.
- Dog rose beneficial effects: improves peripheral circulation, reduces atherosclerosis, respiratory and urinary infections, rheumatism, gout, gall bladder disorders, kidney diseases, general tonic.
- Use organic raw honey and dog rose.
- Use in 1-month cure, then pause for 10 days.

Precautions:

- Dog rose contraindications: avoid use during pregnancy or lactation.
- Do not use if you are allergic to any ingredient
- Contact your doctor with any questions or concerns

Disclaimer: This does not replace medical advice. Check With Your Doctor for symptoms or worsening of condition.

Recipe 51 - Honey and Watermelon Rind

Difficulty: ++; Time: 1 day;

Ingredients:

- 300 g honey
- 500 g watermelon rind

Preparation: Mix honey with grated watermelon rind, put mixture in dark recipients and store them in the fridge. Macerate for 1 day.

How to take it: 1 tablespoon 3 times a day, during meals.

Tips:

- Watermelon properties: contains vitamins (A, B complex, C, D, E), minerals (calcium, magnesium, copper, manganese, potassium, selenium, zinc), choline, flavonoids (lycopene, betaine carotenoids), triterpenoids, amino acids (citrulline: converts into arginine in the body), cucurbitacin E, fiber; anti-oxidant, anti-inflammatory, diuretic, lowers high blood pressure, helps with weight loss, laxative, helps to eliminate gall or kidney stones

- Watermelon beneficial effects: in gall and kidney stones, constipation, prevents heart disorders, boosts immune system, prevents macular degeneration; in high blood pressure, rheumatism, gout, in skin conditions (allergies, dermatitis).
- Use organic raw honey and watermelon.
- Use regularly for better effects

Precautions:

- Do not use if you are allergic to any ingredient.
- Contact your doctor with any questions or concerns

Disclaimer: This does not replace medical advice. Check With Your Doctor for symptoms or worsening of condition.

Constipation

Constipation refers to hard to pass stools and/or infrequent bowel movements. Generally, constipation is depicted as fewer than three passages of stool per week. When the condition persists more than several weeks, it is described as chronic constipation.

Symptoms:

- straining with stool passage +/- pain
- feeling of partial bowel evacuation and of a blockage preventing the passage in the rectum
- hard or lumpy stools
- abdominal pain
- bloating

Seek medical advice if there are unexplained and repeated changes in the bowel habits

Risk factors:

- low-fiber diet, inadequate liquid intake
- lack of or insufficient physical activity
- depression or eating disorder
- drugs: opioids, antidepressants (tricyclic), anticonvulsants, diuretics, antihistamines, anti-arrhytmics, ondansetron, aluminium antacids, some calcium channel blockers (verapamil, nifedipin), iron and calcium supplements.

Recipe 52 - Honey and Liquorice

Difficulty: +; Time: 30 minutes;

Ingredients:

- 2 tablespoons honey
- 1/2 teaspoon chopped liquorice root
- 250 ml water

Preparation: Put liquorice in boiling water and let it infuse and cool. Filter it, then mix with honey.

How to take it: Drink 1/2 amount 30 minutes before meal in the morning and before lunch.

Tips:

- Liquorice properties: contains vitamins (B complex, E), minerals (calcium, magnesium, phosphorous, silicon, iron, zinc, selenium), flavonoids (beta-carotene, quercetin), phenol, glycyrrhizin, thymol, glabridin, phytoestrogens; anti-oxidant, anti-inflammatory, expectorant, growth inhibition of *Helicobacter pylori,* anti-tumor, anti-microbial (also anti-Mycobacterial, antiviral), boosts immunity, lowers cholesterol.

- Liquorice beneficial effects: mouth aphtous ulcers, dyspepsia, gastric and duodenal ulcer associated with *Helicobacter pylori*, liver protection, rheumatism, gout, polyarthritis rheumatoides, menopause, pre-menstrual syndrome, chronic fatigue syndrome, pulmonary infections, pulmonary tuberculosis, acne, shingles, helps in HIV infection, prevention and treatment of cardio-vascular diseases.
- Use organic raw honey and liquorice.

Precautions:

- Liquorice should not be administered during pregnancy, while under digitalis or steroids treatment or in case of renal dysfunction with impaired salt excretion. During the cure, a low salt diet is recommended. May cause body fatigue, kidney disorders, irregular menstruation, may interact with diuretics. Prolonged use may cause the retention of fluid in the body, high blood pressure, low blood potassium levels (hypokalemia), and cataracts. Use in 4 to 6-week cure, followed by 2 to 3-week pause.
- Do not use if you are allergic to any ingredient
- Contact your doctor with any questions or concerns

Disclaimer: This does not replace medical advice. Check With Your Doctor for symptoms or worsening of condition.

Recipe 53 - Honey, Walnuts and Aloe

Difficulty: ++; Time: 15 minutes;

Ingredients:

- 300 g honey
- 200 g walnuts
- 100 g aloe

Preparation: Blend aloe and walnuts, then mix with honey. Store in the fridge.

How to take it: 1 tablespoon 30 minutes before meals, 3 times a day.

Tips:

- Walnuts properties: vitamins (A, B complex, E), minerals (magnesium, zinc, manganese, molybdenum, copper, iron), flavonoids (beta-carotene, lutein, zeaxanthin), proteins (contain L-arginine, which is an essential amino acid); anti-oxidant, anti-inflammatory, lower cholesterol, increase insulin production, laxative.
- Walnuts beneficial effects: prevention of cardio-vascular diseases, lower blood pressure, prevent macular degeneration and cataract, asthma, rheumatoid arthritis, psoriasis, eczema,

improve depression, prevent gallstones, constipation, Type 2 diabetes, great for hair and skin.
- Aloe properties: contains vitamins (A, B9, 12, C), minerals (calcium, magnesium, copper, zinc, phosphorous, manganese, selenium, chromium), phytosterols, phenols (aloin, emodin), hormones (auxins, gibberellins), enzymes (aliiase, bradykinase, alkaline phosphatase, amylase), salicylic acid; anti-inflammatory, anti-microbial, lowers cholesterol, boosts immunity, anti-cancer, analgesic, helps with cough, laxative.
- Aloe beneficial effects: skin disorders (acne, psoriasis, eczema, burns, wounds), genital herpes, dental conditions, gum diseases, mouth ulcers, high blood pressure, sinusitis, respiratory infections, asthma, colitis, irritable bowel disease, gastro-duodenal ulcer, viral hepatitis, malabsorbtion, constipation, adjuvant in diabetes, weight-loss.
- Use organic raw honey, walnuts and aloe
- Use for 1 month for better effects

Precautions:

- Walnuts: may trigger allergy, even anaphylaxis; when used on skin may cause rash; may cause loose stools.
- Aloe may lead rarely to constipation. Caution is advocated in those with liver, gall bladder and kidney conditions. May cause abdominal pains. Avoid in severe, sudden abdominal pain (possible acute appendicitis, bowel occlusion etc.). Avoid in pregnancy, breast feeding women. Do

not combine with steroids (corticosteroids), digoxin, other antiarrhytmics, diuretics. If you are on anticoagulants (blood thinners), ask your doctor before starting a cure!!!
- Do not use if you are allergic to any ingredient
- Contact your doctor with any questions or concerns

Disclaimer: This does not replace medical advice. Check With Your Doctor for symptoms or worsening of condition.

Obesity

Obesity represents a complex condition involving an excessive volume of body fat. It can lead to metabolic syndrome, a plethora of comorbidities consisting of high blood cholesterol and triglycerides, high blood pressure, and type 2 diabetes mellitus.

Diagnostic criteria: body mass index (BMI) ≥ 30.

Body mass index = Weight (kg)/height squared (m^2)

A BMI less than 18.5 means an underweight person. Between 18.5 and 24.9 are the normal values. A BMI from 25.0 to 29.9 signifies an overweight person. In obesity class I BMI is between 30.0 and 34.9, in obesity class II is 35.0 to 39.9, and in extreme obesity (class III) the BMI is over 40.

Risk factors:

- family lifestyle, with referral to eating habits and unhealthy diet, lack of or insufficient physical activity, lack of sleep, and social and economic conditions
- relatives with obesity
- quitting smoking
- pregnancy

- medical conditions (arthritis, hypothyroidism, Cushing syndrome etc.)
- drugs (antidepressants, diabetes, steroids, anticonvulsants, antipsychotic, beta-blockers etc.)

Recipe 54 - Honey, Lemon and Cinnamon

Difficulty: +; Time: 10 minutes;

Ingredients:

- 1 tablespoon honey
- 1 teaspoon cinnamon
- 2 teaspoons lemon juice
- 250 ml warm water

Preparation: Mix honey with cinnamon, lemon juice and water.

How to take it: In the morning before breakfast.

Tips:

- Cinnamon properties: contains vitamins (A, B complex, C), minerals (calcium, iron, manganese, phosphorous), essential oils (cinnamaldehyde, cinnamyl alcohol, cinnamyl acetate), flavonoids (alpha- and beta-carotens, lutein, zeaxanthin, cryptoxanthin, lycopene); anti-oxidant, anti-inflammatory, antimicrobial, antifungal, analgesic, anti-spastic, anti-parasites, haemostatic, peripheral vasodilator, lowers cholesterol, reduces stress and fatigue, promotes healing, anti-cancer.

- Cinnamon beneficial effects: infections (respiratory, gynecological: leucorrhea, vaginitis; digestive: gingivitis, mouth ulcers, enterocolitis, amoebiasis), dyspepsia, GERD, gastritis, peptic ulcer, asthenia, depression, Alzheimer, regulates menstruation, eczema, helps with weight-loss.
- Lemon properties: contains vitamins (A, B complex, C, E), minerals (calcium, magnesium, potassium, copper, manganese, zinc, iron), flavonoids (naringin, naringenin, hesperetin, alfa- and beta-carotenes, lutein, zeaxanthin, beta-cryptoxanthin, tannins), terpenes, citric acid, fibers; anti-oxidant, anti-inflammatory, anti-bacterial, antifungal, antiseptic, immune system booster.
- Lemon beneficial effects: dyspepsia, constipation, respiratory infections, asthma, rheumatism, arthritis, lowers blood pressure, helps with weight-loss, anti-cancer, acne, eczema, burns.
- Use organic raw honey, cinnamon and lemon.
- Use regularly for better effects

Precautions:

- Lemon may cause photosensitivity when used on skin
- Cinnamon: not to be used in pregnancy and in breast-feeding women.
- Do not use if you are allergic to any ingredient
- Contact your doctor with any questions or concerns

Disclaimer: This does not replace medical advice. Check With Your Doctor for symptoms or worsening of condition.

Recipe 55 - Honey and Beer Yeast

Difficulty: +; Time: 10 minutes;

Ingredients:
- 1 tablespoon honey
- 1 teaspoon dried beer yeast
- 600 ml fresh apple juice

Preparation: Mix honey with yeast and apple juice. Store in the fridge. Prepare it every day.

How to take it: 200 ml of the beverage, 3 times a day, 1 hour before meals.

Tips:
- Beer yeast properties: contains vitamins (B complex), minerals (potassium, magnesium, selenium, zinc, copper, iron), beta-1,3 glucan, glutathione, mannan, trehalose; improves blood circulation, balances blood pressure and cholesterol, boosts immunity, anti-aging, helps with calcium storage, prevents constipation, helps with weight-loss, tonic, enhances concentration, decreases fatigue.

- Beer yeast beneficial effects: cardio-vascular diseases, peripheral artheriopathy, metabolic regulation, psoriasis, acne, seborrhea, alopecia, stomatitis, infections, neuro-psychiatric disorders (Alzheimer, Parkinson, dementia), osteoporosis, andropause, and menopause.
- Use organic raw honey and beer yeast.
- Use for 10-30 days, pause for 1 week, then may repeat.

Precautions:

- Do not use if you are allergic to any ingredient
- Contact your doctor with any questions or concerns

Disclaimer: This does not replace medical advice. Check With Your Doctor for symptoms or worsening of condition.

Recipe 56 - Honey and Dill Seeds

Difficulty: +; Time: 15 minutes;

Ingredients:

- 200 g honey
- 4 tablespoons dill seeds

Preparation: Ground the dill seeds in the coffee grinder, then mix with honey. Store in the fridge.

How to take it: In the morning, 30 minutes before meal, 1 tablespoon mixed in 1 glass of water.

Tips:

- Dill properties: contains vitamins (A, B complex, C), minerals (potassium, calcium, magnesium, phosphorous, manganese), flavonoids (beta-carotene equivalents); anti-inflammatory, diuretic, antispastic, lowers cholesterol, estrogenic, stimulates and balances the female hormonal activity, triggers menstruation, stimulates lactate production.
- Dill beneficial effects: high blood pressure, adjuvant in amenorrhea, reduced milk secretion, dysmenorrhea (irregular and painful mentruation), female sterility, premature menopause,

mammary hypoplasia (small breasts), dyspepsia, flatulence (fermentation colitis), gall bladder dyskinesia, urinary infections, helps with weight-loss.
- Use organic raw honey and dill seeds.
- Use regularly for better effects

Precautions:

- Dill contraindications: pregnancy, hyperestrogenism, hypermenorrhea, ovarian cysts, mammary nodules, mammary and genital tumors.
- Do not use if you are allergic to any ingredient
- Contact your doctor with any questions or concerns

Disclaimer: This does not replace medical advice. Check With Your Doctor for symptoms or worsening of condition.

Chapter 7

Kidney Diseases

Urinary Tract Infections

Urinary tract infections refer to infections affecting any part of the urinary system (urethra, bladder, ureters, kidneys). Bladder infections (cystitis) and urethra infections are most frequent. The most frequent cause of infection is *Escherichia coli*.

Symptoms and signs:

- pain: burning sensation with urination in urethral infection, or plain painful urination and discomfort in the lower abdomen in bladder infection; side and upper back pain in kidney infection.
- strong, continuous urinating urge and passing small and numerous amounts of urine in bladder infection
- red urine or with blood cloths
- high fever with shaking and chills, nausea and vomiting in kidney infection

Seek medical advice when experiencing the above-mentioned symptoms.

Risk factors:

- female gender
- large prostate
- abnormalities of the urinary tract
- kidney stones
- catheter use
- recent urinary surgery or investigations
- spinal cord injuries, diabetes, etc.

Recipe 57 - Honey, Garlic and Apple Cider Vinegar

Difficulty: +; Time: 1 week maceration;

Ingredients:

- 200 g honey
- 4 garlic cloves
- 150 ml apple cider vinegar

Preparation: Mix honey with crushed cloves to make a paste, then add apple cider vinegar and stir well. Store in the fridge for 7 days, stir it daily.

How to take it: 1 tablespoon mixed with 1 glass water, 3 times a day, 30 minutes before meals.

Tips:

- Garlic properties: contains vitamins (A, B complex, C, K), minerals (calcium, magnesium, iron, manganese, potassium, selenium, zinc, phosphorous), thiosulfinates (allicin, methyl allyl sulfinates), ajoenes, sulfides, sulfoxides (alliin, isoalliin, methiin, garlicins), flavonoids (beta-carotene, lutein, zeaxanthin); anti-bacterial, anti-viral, anti-fungal, anti-inflammatory, anti-oxidant, anti-

platelet activity, decreases cholesterol, lowers blood sugar, lowers blood pressure.
- Garlic beneficial effects: heart diseases, high blood pressure, various cancers, respiratory infections, sinusitis, asthma, gastric and duodenal ulcers, especially associated with *Helicobacter pylori*, liver cirrhosis, osteoporosis, improves performance and reduces fatigue, detoxifies the body of heavy metals.
- Apple cider vinegar properties: contains vitamins (B complex, C, folate, pantothenic acid), minerals (calcium, potassium, sodium, iron, phosphorus), acetic acid, malic acid, pectin, polyphenols (flavonols, flavanols, tannins, anthocyanins, dihydrochalcones, hydroxycinnamic acids); boosts immunity, anti-microbial, anti-inflammatory, antioxidant, lowers cholesterol, lowers blood sugar, acts as anti-acid.
- Apple cider vinegar beneficial effects: in infections (sinusitis, sore throat, asthma, other respiratory infections, urinary tract infections, etc), allergies, arthritis, gout, cardiovascular diseases, improves digestion, prevents constipation, helps with weight loss, in skin conditions (acne, eczema).
- Use organic raw honey, garlic and apple cider vinegar.
- Use regularly for better effects

Precautions:

- Garlic: may lower Saquinavir levels and may interact with some anticoagulants and diabetes medication. If you are on anticoagulants (blood thinners), ask your doctor before starting a cure!!! May cause flatulence and nausea. Locally applied may lead to irritation, urticaria, anaphylaxis.
- Do not use if you are allergic to any ingredient
- Contact your doctor with any questions or concerns

Disclaimer: This does not replace medical advice. Check With Your Doctor for symptoms or worsening of condition.

Recipe 58 - Honey, Lemon, Olive Oil, and Parsley Root

Difficulty: ++; Time: 30 minutes;

Ingredients:

- 6 tablespoons honey
- 60 g parsley root
- 4 tablespoons olive oil
- 1 medium lemon

Preparation: Mix grated parsley root in a blender with lemon, honey and olive oil. Store the mixture in a sealed jar in the fridge.

How to take it: 1 tablespoon, in the morning before breakfast.

Tips:

- Lemon properties: contains vitamins (A, B complex, C, E), minerals (calcium, magnesium, potassium, copper, manganese, zinc, iron), flavonoids (naringin, naringenin, hesperetin, alfa- and beta-carotenes, lutein, zeaxanthin, beta-cryptoxanthin, tannins), terpenes, citric acid, fibers; anti-oxidant, anti-inflammatory, anti-bacterial, antifungal, antiseptic, immune system booster.

- Lemon beneficial effects: dyspepsia, constipation, respiratory infections, asthma, rheumatism, arthritis, lowers blood pressure, helps with weight-loss, anti-cancer, acne, eczema, burns.
- Olive oil properties: contains vitamins (E, K), fatty acids (high content of oleic acid, omega-3, omega-6), flavonoids: flavonols (kaempferol, quercetin), flavones (luteolin, apigenin), anthocyanidins (peonidins, cyanidins), as well as tyrosols (tyrosol, hydroxytyrosol, oleuropein), secoiridoids (oleuropein), hydroxybenzoic acids (syringic acid, vanillic acid), hydroxycinnamic acids (coumaric acid, caffeic acid, ferulic acid, cinnamic acid), lignans (pinoresinol); lowers blood pressure, lowers cholesterol, anti-oxidant, antimicrobial (including *Helicobacter pylori*), anti-inflammatory, promotes bone formation.
- Olive oil beneficial effects: heart diseases, diabetes, osteoporosis, anti-cancer, respiratory infections, stomach and duodenal ulcer (especially associated with *Helicobacter pylori*), weight-loss.
- Parsley properties: contains vitamins (A, B complex, C-high content, K, E), minerals (calcium, magnesium, iron, potassium, sodium, phosphorous), flavonoids (beta-carotene), essential fatty acids, carbohydrates, volatile oils, apiole (natural estrogen); anti-oxidant, anti-bacterial, diuretic, lowers cholesterol, helps dissolve gall stones, stimulates uterine contractions and diminishes milk secretion, boosts immune system.
- Parsley beneficial effects: infections, high blood pressure, blood flow disturbances, meteor-

ism and abdominal colics, amenorrhea, pre-menstrual syndrome, menopause, anorexia, fatigue, edema treatment, healing wounds, conjunctivitis, liver disturbances (cirrhosis, hepatitis), anemia, gout.

- Use organic raw honey, lemon, parsley and olive oil.
- Use for 10 days for better effects.

Precautions:

- Lemon may cause photosensitivity when used on skin
- Parsley: contraindicated in pregnancy and breastfeeding.
- Do not use if you are allergic to any ingredient
- Contact your doctor with any questions or concerns

Disclaimer: This does not replace medical advice. Check With Your Doctor for symptoms or worsening of condition.

Recipe 59 - Honey, Lemon and Carrot Juice

Difficulty: +; Time: 10 minutes;

Ingredients:

- 1 tablespoon honey
- 125 ml fresh lemon juice
- 125 ml fresh carrot juice

Preparation: Mix honey with the juices.

How to take it: 3 times a day, 30 minutes before meals.

Tips:

- Lemon properties: contains vitamins (A, B complex, C, E), minerals (calcium, magnesium, potassium, copper, manganese, zinc, iron), flavonoids (naringin, naringenin, hesperetin, alfa- and beta-carotenes, lutein, zeaxanthin, beta-cryptoxanthin, tannins), terpenes, citric acid, fibers; anti-oxidant, anti-inflammatory, anti-bacterial, antifungal, antiseptic, immune system booster.
- Lemon beneficial effects: dyspepsia, constipation, respiratory infections, asthma, rheumatism, arthritis, lowers blood pressure, helps with weight-loss, anti-cancer, acne, eczema, burns.

- Carrot properties: contains vitamins (A, B complex, C, E, K), minerals (copper, manganese, molybdenum), carotenoids (alfa- and beta-caroten, lutein), anthocyanindins, hydroxycinamic acid, high fiber content; anti-oxidant, anti-inflammatory, antibacterial, detoxifying, lowers cholesterol, lowers insulin resistance, boosts immunity.
- Carrot beneficial effects: prevents macular degeneration, improves vision, prevents heart disease, stroke, helps with gum and teeth disorders, improves digestion, anti-cancer.
- Use organic raw honey, lemon and carrot juice.
- Use 7 days for better effects.

Precautions:

- Lemon may cause photosensitivity when used on skin
- Consumed in excess, carrots may color the skin orange (face, palms, feet). Avoid in small intestine inflammation, acute gastro-duodenal ulcer.
- Do not use if you are allergic to any ingredient
- Contact your doctor with any questions or concerns

Disclaimer: This does not replace medical advice. Check With Your Doctor for symptoms or worsening of condition.

Recipe 60 - Honey, Apple and Dog Rose Juice

Difficulty: +; Time: 10 minutes;

Ingredients:

- 1 teaspoon honey
- 125 ml fresh apple juice
- 125 ml fresh dog rose juice

Preparation: Mix honey with juices.

How to take it: 3 times a day, 30 minutes before meals.

Tips:

- Apple properties: contains vitamins (A, B complex, C, E, PP), minerals (calcium, magnesium, iodine, iron, silicon, molybdenum, phosphorous), flavonoids (quercetin, kaempferol, myricetin, anthocyanins, epicatechin), chlorogenic acid, triterpenoids, fiber (high content); expectorant, anti-microbial, anti-oxidant, regulates cholesterol.
- Apple beneficial effects: infections, stress, depression, fatigue, colitis, billiary diskinesia, constipation, improves hemorrhoids, helps with weight-loss, rheumatism, gout, prevents cardiovascular disorders, wounds healing, burns, eczema, acne.

- Dog rose properties: contains vitamins (A, B complex, C - high amounts, E, F), minerals (magnesium, calcium, manganese, selenium, iron, zinc, phosphorous, sulfur), flavonoids (carotenoids, tannins), terpenoids, organic acids; reduces small blood vessels fragility, anti-oxidant, anti-inflammatory, lowers blood sugar, boosts immunity, promotes regeneration, diuretic, stimulates uric acid removal.
- Dog rose beneficial effects: improves peripheral circulation, reduces atherosclerosis, respiratory and urinary infections, rheumatism, gout, gall bladder disorders, kidney diseases, general tonic.
- Use organic raw honey, apple and dog rose juice.
- Use 7 days for better effects.

Precautions:

- Dog rose contraindications: avoid use during pregnancy or lactation.
- Do not use if you are allergic to any ingredient
- Contact your doctor with any questions or concerns

Disclaimer: This does not replace medical advice. Check With Your Doctor for symptoms or worsening of condition.

Recipe 61 - Honey and Celery Seeds

Difficulty: ++; Time: 8 hours;

Ingredients:

- 600 g honey
- 5 tablespoons celery seeds

Preparation: Put crushed celery seeds in 100 ml lukewarm water and let them macerate 8 hours in the fridge. Mix in the honey.

How to take it: 2 teaspoons in the morning, 30 minutes before meal.

Tips:

- Celery properties: contains vitamins (A, B complex, C), minerals (calcium, magnesium, potassium, sodium, iron, zinc, phosphorous, etc), flavonoids (beta-caroten, lutein, zeaxanthin), essential oils (apiol, sedanolide), furanocoumarins (psoralen, bergapten), linoleic acid, lunularin, flavonols (quercetin, kampferol), terpenes, 3-n-butylphtalide; anti-oxidant, anti-inflammatory, anti-microbial, stimulates digestion, diuretic, expectorant, lowers cholesterol, calming effect.
- Celery beneficial effects: kidney infections and stones, lowers high blood pressure, respiratory infections (asthma, bronchitis), helps with stress,

arthritis, rheumatism, gout, in mouth ulcers, gingivitis, helps with gastro-duodenal ulcers, liver detoxification, constipation, helps with weight-loss, diabetes, skin wounds.
- Use organic raw honey and celery seeds.
- Use 1 month for better effects.

Precautions:

- Celery: may cause allergy and photosensibilisation. Avoid in pregnancy. If you are on anticoagulants (blood thinners), ask your doctor before starting a cure!!!
- Do not use if you are allergic to any ingredient
- Contact your doctor with any questions or concerns

Disclaimer: This does not replace medical advice. Check With Your Doctor for symptoms or worsening of condition.

Recipe 62 - Honey and Dog Rose Seeds

Difficulty: ++; Time: 12 hours;

Ingredients:

- 2 tablespoons honey
- 2 tablespoons dog rose seeds
- 500 ml water

Preparation: Macerate 2 tablespoons dog rose seeds in 250 ml water for 10 hours, then filter it. Boil the filtered plant residue in another 250-ml water for 15 minutes and let it cool. Mix the two solutions, add honey and stir thoroughly. Store in the fridge.

How to take it: 250 ml twice a day, 30 minutes before meals.

Tips:

- Dog rose properties: contains vitamins (A, B complex, C - high amounts, E, F), minerals (magnesium, calcium, manganese, selenium, iron, zinc, phosphorous, sulfur), flavonoids (carotenoids, tannins), terpenoids, organic acids; reduces small blood vessels fragility, anti-oxidant, anti-inflam-

matory, lowers blood sugar, boosts immunity, promotes regeneration, diuretic, stimulates uric acid removal.
- Dog rose beneficial effects: improves peripheral circulation, reduces atherosclerosis, respiratory and urinary infections, rheumatism, gout, gall bladder disorders, kidney diseases, general tonic.
- Use organic raw honey and dog rose.
- Use in 2-week cure, then pause for 2 weeks.

Precautions:

- Dog rose contraindications: avoid use during pregnancy or lactation.
- Do not use if you are allergic to any ingredient
- Contact your doctor with any questions or concerns

Disclaimer: This does not replace medical advice. Check With Your Doctor for symptoms or worsening of condition.

Renal Lithiasis (Kidney Stones)

Renal lithiasis is a condition in which inside the urinary system solid deposits of salts and minerals are formed. Usually, they are eliminated via the urine stream, but, sometimes, they may become blocked in the urinary tract, leading to urinary infections or other complications, which may require surgery. In some cases, the patients are asymptomatic.

Symptoms:

- pain on urination; pain radiating to the lower abdomen and groin; excruciating pain in the side and below the ribs, in the back.
- incessant need to urinate, passing of small amounts of urine, more often than usual
- pink or red urine, cloudy
- fever, chills, nausea and vomiting, if complicated by infection.

Seek medical advice if severe pain, if pain accompanied by fever, chills, nausea and vomiting, or in case off difficulty passing urine and presence of blood in urine.

Risk factors:

- dietary habits: diet with high content in protein, sugar, salt, insufficient hydration
- obesity
- relatives with kidney stones
- digestive conditions and surgery (Crohn's disease, chronic diarrhea, gastric bypass surgery, etc.)
- other diseases (hyperparathyroidism, primary hyperoxaluria, renal tubular acidosis, medullary sponge kidney).

Recipe 63 - Honey, Elderberry Flowers, and Lemon

Difficulty: ++; Time: 4 days;

Ingredients:

- 350 g honey
- 5 tablespoons fresh chopped elderberry flowers
- 3 lemons
- 5-liter water

Preparation: Mix honey with elderberry flowers, juice from the lemons and water in a large glass jar. Seal the jar and let the mixture ferment for 3-4 days. Stir twice a day with a wooden spoon. After 4 days, filter the liquid and store in 1 liter glass bottles in the fridge.

How to take it: 1 liter daily for 10-14 days, every 3 months.

Tips:

- Elderberry flowers properties: vitamins (A, B complex, C), minerals (calcium, potassium, phosphorous, iron, manganese), tannins, sterols,

sugars (among which cyanogenic glycosides), flavonoids (quercetin, beta-carotene), fatty acids; anti-oxidant, lower cholesterol, anti-inflammatory, expectorant, astringent, boost immunity, diuretic, mild laxative.
- Elderberry flowers beneficial effects: lower blood pressure, respiratory infections, asthma, sinusitis, sore throat, ear infections, skin infections (acne, boils, skin rashes), rheumatism, arthritis, gout; help with kidney stones, constipation.
- Lemon properties: contains vitamins (A, B complex, C, E), minerals (calcium, magnesium, potassium, copper, manganese, zinc, iron), flavonoids (naringin, naringenin, hesperetin, alfa- and beta-carotenes, lutein, zeaxanthin, beta-cryptoxanthin, tannins), terpenes, citric acid, fibers; anti-oxidant, anti-inflammatory, anti-bacterial, antifungal, antiseptic, immune system booster.
- Lemon beneficial effects: dyspepsia, constipation, respiratory infections, asthma, rheumatism, arthritis, lowers blood pressure, helps with weight-loss, anti-cancer, acne, eczema, burns.
- Use organic raw honey, lemons and elderberry flowers.
- Use regularly for better effects

Precautions:

- Elderberry: contraindications in acute and chronic diarrhea. In high doses (over 200 g per day), may lead to intoxication (throat irritation, heartburn, nausea and vomiting, trouble breathing, convulsions).

- Lemon may cause photosensitivity when used on skin
- Do not use if you are allergic to any ingredient
- Contact your doctor with any questions or concerns

Disclaimer: This does not replace medical advice. Check With Your Doctor for symptoms or worsening of condition.

Recipe 64 - Honey, Cucumber, Carrot, Black Radish and Red Beets

Difficulty: +; Time: 10 minutes;

Ingredients:

- 3 teaspoons honey
- 150 ml cucumber juice
- 150 ml carrot juice
- 150 ml black radish juice
- 150 ml red beet juice

Preparation: Mix honey with juices.

How to take it: 300 ml 30 minutes before meals, in the morning and at lunch.

Tips:

- Cucumber properties: 95% water, vitamins (A, B complex, C, K), minerals (calcium, magnesium, potassium, iron, phosphorous, molybdenum, selenium, zinc), flavonoids (quercetin, apigenin, kaempherol, alpha- and beta-caroten, lutein, zeaxanthin), triterpenes (cucurbitacin A, B, C, D), lignans (lariciresinol, pinoresinol); stimulates blood circulation, anti-oxidant, anti-inflammatory,

hydrating, diuretic, astringent, dissolves uric acid and urates.
- Cucumber beneficial effects: high blood pressure, gout, arthritis, kidney stones, constipation, helps with weight-loss, detoxification. Skin benefits in acne, dermatitis, sunburns.
- Carrot properties: contains vitamins (A, B complex, C, E, K), minerals (copper, manganese, molybdenum), carotenoids (alfa- and beta-caroten, lutein), anthocyanindins, hydroxycinamic acid, high fiber content; anti-oxidant, anti-inflammatory, antibacterial, detoxifying, lowers cholesterol, lowers insulin resistance, boosts immunity.
- Carrot beneficial effects: prevents macular degeneration, improves vision, prevents heart disease, stroke, helps with gum and teeth disorders, improves digestion, anti-cancer.
- Black radish properties: contains vitamins (C, B complex), minerals (calcium, magnesium, copper, iron), indoles, flavonoids (zeaxanthin, lutein, beta-carotens, anthocyanins), high fiber content; expectorant, anti-congestive, bactericidal, disinfectant, antioxidant, diuretic, lowers body fever, lowers blood pressure, decreases blood sugar, anti-cancer.
- Black radish beneficial effects: respiratory infections (asthma, bronchitis, pneumonia convalescence, sinusitis and sore throats), high blood pressure, constipation, weight loss, diabetes, many types of cancers, in skin disorders.
- Red beets properties: contain vitamins (A, B complex, C, E, K), minerals (calcium, magnesium, copper, manganese), flavonoids (high content

beta-caroten, lutein), high content in carbohydrates, betalains (vulgaxanthin, betanin); anti-oxidant, anti-inflammatory, detoxifying, lower cholesterol.

- Red beets beneficial effects: anemia, help prevent macular degeneration and cataracts, skin conditions, constipation.
- Use organic raw honey, cucumber, carrots, black radish and red beets.
- Use regularly for 1 month for better effects.

Precautions:

- Cucumber contraindications: severe high blood pressure, ascitis, and other conditions with fluid retention.
- Consumed in excess, carrots may color the skin orange (face, palms, feet). Avoid in small intestine inflammation, acute gastro-duodenal ulcer.
- Red beets may cause rarely red or pink-colored urine (beeturia), especially in people with iron deficiency; less commonly color the stools in red. Avoid eating in excess - may induce kidney or gall-bladder stones.
- Do not use if you are allergic to any ingredient
- Contact your doctor with any questions or concerns

Disclaimer: This does not replace medical advice. Check With Your Doctor for symptoms or worsening of condition.

Recipe 65 - Honey and Corn Silk (macerate)

Difficulty: +; Time: 9 hours overnight;

Ingredients:

- 2 tablespoons honey
- 2 tablespoons dried corn silk
- 1 liter water

Preparation: Mix dried corn silk with 500 ml water and let overnight to macerate (9 hours). Filter it in the morning, and put the corn silk in 500 ml boiling water. Let it cool, then filter it, and mix the liquid with the macerate liquid and with the honey.

How to take it: Drink it over the day.

Tips:

- Corn silk properties: contains vitamins (A, B complex, C, E), minerals (magnesium, iron, zinc, potassium, phosphorous), betaine, flavonoids (tannins), alantoine, volatile oils, ergosterine, proteins (zeine, with high content of leucine and glutamic acid), starch; antispastic, diuretic, haemostatic, improves liver function, anti-inflammatory, astringent; in high doses, decreases blood sugar.

- Corn silk beneficial effects: kidney stones, urinary tract infections, prostatitis, cardio-vascular conditions, arthritis, rheumatism, high blood pressure, dysmenorrhea, menopause, edema, ascitis, helps with weight-loss.
- Use organic raw honey and corn silk.
- Use regularly for 1 week for better effects. May be repeated after 1 week.

Precautions:

Corn silk: avoid in pregnancy, precaution in diabetes, hypertension (interaction with Captopril, Enalapril, Furosemid), simultaneous administration of anti-inflammatory drugs which lower blood potassium; can reduce the efficacy of warfarin. Seek medical advice before starting the treatment.

- Do not use if you are allergic to any ingredient
- Contact your doctor with any questions or concerns

Disclaimer: This does not replace medical advice. Check With Your Doctor for symptoms or worsening of condition.

Recipe 66 - Honey and Corn Silk (infusion)

Difficulty: +; Time: 30 minutes;

Ingredients:

- 1 teaspoon honey
- 1 teaspoon dried corn silk
- 250 ml water

Preparation: Infuse dried corn silk with 250 ml boiling water for 2 minutes, then filter it and let it cool. Mix it with honey.

How to take it: 2 to 3 cups per day, 30 minutes before meals.

Tips:

- Corn silk properties: contains vitamins (A, B complex, C, E), minerals (magnesium, iron, zinc, potassium, phosphorous), betaine, flavonoids (tannins), alantoine, volatile oils, ergosterine, proteins (zeine, with high content of leucine and glutamic acid), starch; antispastic, diuretic, haemostatic, improves liver function, anti-inflammatory, astringent; in high doses, decreases blood sugar.
- Corn silk beneficial effects: kidney stones, urinary tract infections, prostatitis, cardio-vascular

conditions, arthritis, rheumatism, high blood pressure, dysmenorrhea, menopause, edema, ascitis, helps with weight-loss.
- Use organic raw honey and corn silk.
- Use regularly for 1 week for better effects. May be repeated after 1 week.

Precautions:

Corn silk: avoid in pregnancy, precaution in diabetes, hypertension (interaction with Captopril, Enalapril, Furosemid), simultaneous administration of anti-inflammatory drugs which lower blood potassium; can reduce the efficacy of warfarin. Seek medical advice before starting the treatment.

- Do not use if you are allergic to any ingredient
- Contact your doctor with any questions or concerns

Disclaimer: This does not replace medical advice. Check With Your Doctor for symptoms or worsening of condition.

Recipe 67 - Honey and Corn Silk (decoction)

Difficulty: +; Time: 30 minutes;

Ingredients:

- 5 teaspoons honey
- 5 tablespoons dried corn silk
- 1 liter water

Preparation: Boil dried corn silk with 1 liter water for 2 hours at low heat, then filter it and let it cool. Mix it with honey.

How to take it: Drink it over the day.

Tips:

- Corn silk properties: contains vitamins (A, B complex, C, E), minerals (magnesium, iron, zinc, potassium, phosphorous), betaine, flavonoids (tannins), alantoine, volatile oils, ergosterine, proteins (zeine, with high content of leucine and glutamic acid), starch; antispastic, diuretic, haemostatic, improves liver function, anti-inflammatory, astringent; in high doses, decreases blood sugar.
- Corn silk beneficial effects: kidney stones, urinary tract infections, prostatitis, cardio-vascular

conditions, arthritis, rheumatism, high blood pressure, dysmenorrhea, menopause, edema, ascitis, helps with weight-loss.
- Use organic raw honey and corn silk.
- Use regularly for 1 week for better effects. May be repeated after 1 week.

Precautions:

Corn silk: avoid in pregnancy, precaution in diabetes, hypertension (interaction with Captopril, Enalapril, Furosemid), simultaneous administration of anti-inflammatory drugs which lower blood potassium; can reduce the efficacy of Warfarin. Seek medical advice before starting the treatment.

- Do not use if you are allergic to any ingredient
- Contact your doctor with any questions or concerns

Disclaimer: This does not replace medical advice. Check With Your Doctor for symptoms or worsening of condition.

Recipe 68 - Honey and Green Walnuts

Difficulty: ++; Time: 1 month;

Ingredients:

- 500 g honey
- 200 g green walnuts

Preparation: Mix honey with chopped green walnuts, put mixture in a sealed jar, and store them in a sunny place for a month. Stir every 2-3 days with a wooden spoon. After 1 month store in a dark place.

How to take it: 1 tablespoon in the morning before breakfast.

Tips:

- Walnuts properties: vitamins (A, B complex, E), minerals (magnesium, zinc, manganese, molybdenum, copper, iron), flavonoids (beta-carotene, lutein, zeaxanthin), proteins (contain L-arginine, which is an essential amino acid); anti-oxidant, anti-inflammatory, lower cholesterol, increase insulin production, laxative.
- Walnuts beneficial effects: prevention of cardio-vascular diseases, lower blood pressure,

prevent macular degeneration and cataract, asthma, rheumatoid arthritis, psoriasis, eczema, improve depression, prevent gallstones, constipation, Type 2 diabetes, great for hair and skin.
- Use organic raw honey and green walnuts.

Precautions:

- Walnuts: may trigger allergy, even anaphylaxis; when used on skin may cause rash; may cause loose stools.
- Do not use if you are allergic to any ingredient
- Contact your doctor with any questions or concerns

Disclaimer: This does not replace medical advice. Check With Your Doctor for symptoms or worsening of condition.

Benign Prostatic Hyperplasia (Prostate Gland Enlargement)

Prostate gland enlargement is a frequent condition in aging men, which can cause resistance to, or even block the urinary flow out of the bladder. The symptomatology of the condition worsens progressively over time.

Symptoms:

- Increased frequency and urgency of urination, including during nighttime
- strenuous starting urination
- struggling during urination
- intermittent and weak urine stream, with dribbling in the end
- incapacity of completely emptying of the bladder
- presence of blood in the urine, rarely

Seek medical advice when experiencing the above-mentioned symptoms

Risk factors:

- aging
- lifestyle (obesity, lack of physical exercise)
- relatives with prostate hyperplasia
- diseases (diabetes, heart disease)

Recipe 69 - Honey and Pumpkin Seeds

Difficulty: ++; Time: 7 days;

Ingredients:

- 750 g honey
- 750 g fresh pumpkin seeds

Preparation: Mix honey with pumpkinseeds. Put them in a closed jar and let them macerate for 1 week in the fridge. Store in the fridge.

How to take it: 1 teaspoon, 30 minutes before meals in the morning and in the evening.

Tips:

- Pumpkin seeds properties: contain vitamins (A, B complex, C, E), minerals (zinc, magnesium, manganese, phosphorous, iron, copper), flavonoids (alpha- and beta-carotene, cryptoxanthin, lutein, zeaxanthin), proteins, phenolic acids (hydroxybenzoic, caffeic, syringic, coumaric, sinapic, vanillic, protocatechuic, ferulic), lignans (pinoresinol, lariciresinol, medioresinol), phytosterols (beta-sitosterol, avenasterol, sitostanol); antioxidant, anti-bacterial, anti-viral, anti-fungal, anti-cancer, general tonic.

- Pumpkin seeds beneficial effects: various infections, diabetes, prostate benign enlargement.
- Use organic raw honey and pumpkin seeds.
- Use regularly for better effects

Precautions:

- Do not use if you are allergic to any ingredient
- Contact your doctor with any questions or concerns

Disclaimer: This does not replace medical advice. Check With Your Doctor for symptoms or worsening of condition.

Recipe 70 - Honey, Horseradish and Lemon

Difficulty: ++; Time: 15 minutes;

Ingredients:

- 100 g honey
- 100 g horseradish
- 50 ml lemon juice

Preparation: Mix honey with grated horseradish and lemon juice. Store the mixture in the fridge.

How to take it: 1 tablespoon 3 times a day, 30 minutes before meals.

Tips:

- Horseradish properties: contains vitamins (A, B complex, C - high content), minerals (calcium, magnesium, iron, phosphorous, zinc, copper, manganese), flavonoids (beta-carotene, lutein, zeaxanthin) glutamines, asparagine, sinigrin (a glucosinolate), allyl isothiocyanate; cardiotonic, anti-oxidant, anti-inflammatory, relaxant, expectorant, laxative.

- Horseradish beneficial effects: lowers blood pressure, helps in angina pectoris, respiratory infections, cold, sinusitis, bronchitis, asthma, helps in anorexia etc.
- Lemon properties: contains vitamins (A, B complex, C, E), minerals (calcium, magnesium, potassium, copper, manganese, zinc, iron), flavonoids (naringin, naringenin, hesperetin, alfa- and beta-carotenes, lutein, zeaxanthin, beta-cryptoxanthin, tannins), terpenes, citric acid, fibers; anti-oxidant, anti-inflammatory, anti-bacterial, antifungal, antiseptic, immune system booster.
- Lemon beneficial effects: dyspepsia, constipation, respiratory infections, asthma, rheumatism, arthritis, lowers blood pressure, helps with weight-loss, anti-cancer, acne, eczema, burns.
- Use organic raw honey, horseradish and lemon.
- Use regularly for better effects

Precautions:

- Horseradish contraindications: palpitations (cardiac rhythm disturbances), hemorrhoids.
- Lemon may cause photosensitivity when used on skin
- Do not use if you are allergic to any ingredient
- Contact your doctor with any questions or concerns

Disclaimer: This does not replace medical advice. Check With Your Doctor for symptoms or worsening of condition.

Recipe 71 - Honey and Celery Juice

Difficulty: +; Time: 10 minutes;

Ingredients:

- 500 g honey
- 250 ml celery juice

Preparation: Mix honey with celery juice. Store in the fridge.

How to take it: 1 tablespoon 3 times a day, 30 minutes before meals.

Tips:

- Celery properties: contains vitamins (A, B complex, C), minerals (calcium, magnesium, potassium, sodium, iron, zinc, phosphorous, etc), flavonoids (beta-caroten, lutein, zeaxanthin, flavonols: quercetin, kampferol), essential oils (apiol, sedanolide), furanocoumarins (psoralen, bergapten), linoleic acid, lunularin, terpenes, 3-n-butyl-phtalide; anti-oxidant, anti-inflammatory, anti-microbial, stimulates digestion, diuretic, expectorant, lowers cholesterol, calming effect.

- Celery beneficial effects: kidney infections and stones, lowers high blood pressure, respiratory infections (asthma, bronchitis), helps with stress, arthritis, rheumatism, gout, in mouth ulcers, gingivitis, helps with gastro-duodenal ulcers, liver detoxification, constipation, helps with weight-loss, diabetes, skin wounds.
- Use organic raw honey and celery.
- Use regularly for better effects

Precautions:

- Celery: may cause allergy and photosensibilisation. Avoid in pregnancy. If you are on anticoagulants (blood thinners), ask your doctor before starting a cure!!!
- Do not use if you are allergic to any ingredient
- Contact your doctor with any questions or concerns

Disclaimer: This does not replace medical advice. Check With Your Doctor for symptoms or worsening of condition.

Recipe 72 - Honey, Carrots, Walnuts and Turmeric

Difficulty: ++; Time: 30 minutes;

Ingredients:

- 500 g honey
- 250 g carrots
- 150 g walnuts
- 2 teaspoons turmeric

Preparation: Mix honey with grated carrots, crushed walnuts and turmeric. Store in the fridge.

How to take it: 1 teaspoon 3 times a day, 30 minutes before meals.

Tips:

- Carrot properties: contains vitamins (A, B complex, C, E, K), minerals (copper, manganese, molybdenum), carotenoids (alfa- and beta-caroten, lutein), anthocyanindins, hydroxycinamic acid, high fiber content; anti-oxidant, anti-inflammatory, antibacterial, detoxifying, lowers cholesterol, lowers insulin resistance, boosts immunity.

- Carrot beneficial effects: prevents macular degeneration, improves vision, prevents heart disease, stroke, helps with gum and teeth disorders, improves digestion, anti-cancer.
- Walnuts properties: vitamins (A, B complex, E), minerals (magnesium, zinc, manganese, molybdenum, copper, iron), flavonoids (beta-carotene, lutein, zeaxanthin), proteins (contain L-arginine, which is an essential amino acid); anti-oxidant, anti-inflammatory, lower cholesterol, increase insulin production, laxative.
- Walnuts beneficial effects: prevention of cardio-vascular diseases, lower blood pressure, prevent macular degeneration and cataract, asthma, rheumatoid arthritis, psoriasis, eczema, improve depression, prevent gallstones, constipation, Type 2 diabetes, great for hair and skin.
- Turmeric properties: vitamins (B complex, C, E, K), minerals (potassium, calcium, magnesium, copper, phosphorous, zinc, iron, selenium, manganese), curcuminoids (curcumin, demethoxycurcumin), volatile oils (turmerone, zingiberene, atlantone), resins, proteins, sugars; anti-inflammatory, mood improvement, blood thinning, lowers cholesterol, modulation of the immune response, painkiller, in Type 2 Diabetes reduces blood sugar and diminishes insulin resistance, anti-cancer.
- Turmeric beneficial effects: infections, Alzheimer's disease, depression, arthritis, inflammatory digestive tract diseases, cardio-vascular diseases, obesity, psoriasis, autoimmune diseases (lupus, rheumatoid arthritis, etc.).

- Use organic raw honey, carrots, walnuts and turmeric.
- Use regularly for better effects

Precautions:

- Consumed in excess, carrots may color the skin orange (face, palms, feet). Avoid in small intestine inflammation, acute gastro-duodenal ulcer.
- Walnuts: may trigger allergy, even anaphylaxis; when used on skin may cause rash; may cause loose stools.
- Turmeric contraindications: pregnant women, during menstruation. Side-Effects: nausea and diarrhea, lower blood pressure, higher bleeding risk (especially combined with anticoagulants). If you are on anticoagulants (blood thinners), ask your doctor before starting a cure!!!
- Do not use if you are allergic to any ingredient
- Contact your doctor with any questions or concerns

Disclaimer: This does not replace medical advice. Check With Your Doctor for symptoms or worsening of condition.

Chapter 8

Endocrine Diseases

Menopause

Menopause is a natural process occurring in the fifth or sixth decade of age, about one year after the last menstrual period. Just before menopause, periods become irregular, finally stopping altogether.

Symptoms:

- hot flashes and sweats (avoid alcohol, smoking, caffeine)
- mood changes, anxiety, feelings of loss
- sleep problems
- weight gain
- vaginal and skin dryness
- breast changes
- thinner hair

Recipe 73 - Honey and Liquorice (infusion)

Difficulty: +; Time: 30 minutes;

Ingredients:

- 1 tablespoon honey
- 2 teaspoons powder liquorice
- 250 ml water

Preparation: Infuse 2 teaspoons powdered liquorice in 250 ml hot water for 15 minutes, then filter it and let it cool. Mix the solution with honey and stir thoroughly.

How to take it: 1 cup twice a day, 30 minutes before meals, not longer than 1 month.

Tips:

- Liquorice properties: contains vitamins (B complex, E), minerals (calcium, magnesium, phosphorous, silicon, iron, zinc, selenium), flavonoids (beta-carotene, quercetin), phenol, glycyrrhizin, thymol, glabridin, phytoestrogens; anti-oxidant, anti-inflammatory, expectorant, growth inhibition of *Helicobacter pylori,* anti-tumor, anti-microbial (also anti-Mycobacterial, antiviral), boosts immunity, lowers cholesterol.

- Liquorice beneficial effects: mouth aphtous ulcers, dyspepsia, gastric and duodenal ulcer associated with *Helicobacter pylori*, liver protection, rheumatism, gout, polyarthritis rheumatoides, menopause, pre-menstrual syndrome, chronic fatigue syndrome, pulmonary infections, pulmonary tuberculosis, acne, shingles, helps in HIV infection, prevention and treatment of cardio-vascular diseases.
- Use organic raw honey and liquorice.
- Use regularly for better effects

Precautions:

- Liquorice should not be administered during pregnancy, while under digitalis or steroids treatment or in case of renal dysfunction with impaired salt excretion. During the cure, a low salt diet is recommended. May cause body fatigue, kidney disorders, irregular menstruation, may interact with diuretics. Prolonged use may cause the retention of fluid in the body, high blood pressure, low blood potassium levels (hypokalemia), and cataracts.
- Do not use if you are allergic to any ingredient
- Contact your doctor with any questions or concerns

Disclaimer: This does not replace medical advice. Check With Your Doctor for symptoms or worsening of condition.

Recipe 74 - Honey and Hawthorn (infusion)

Difficulty: +; Time: 30 minutes;

Ingredients:
- 1 1/2 teaspoon honey
- 1 tablespoon dried hawthorn
- 250 ml water

Preparation: Infuse 1 tablespoon dried hawthorn in 250 ml boiling water for 20 minutes, then filter it. Mix it with honey.

How to take it: 3 times a day, 30 minutes before meals.

Tips:

- Hawthorn properties: contains vitamins (B, C, E), flavonoids (tannins, epicatechin, quercetin, rutin, C-glycosylated flavone derivative, hyperoside, kaempferol, anthocyanin, anthocyanidins), triterpenes, chlorogenic acids, organic acids (citric, nicotinic, malic), volatile oils; anti-oxidant, anti-inflammatory, sedativ, cardiotonic, cardioprotective, hypolipidaemic, antiarrhytmic, coronary vasodilator, lowers blood pressure.

- Hawthorn beneficial effects: anxiety, depression, migraines, insomnia, high blood pressure, ischemic cardiomyopathie, cardiac insufficiency, palpitations.
- Use organic raw honey and hawthorn.
- Use regularly for better effects

Precautions:

- Hawthorn: avoid in pregnancy. In high dose, it may reduce blood pressure and cause dizziness and faint. May increase the activity of digoxine, beta-blockers, calcium channel blockers, and anti-depressives. If you are on anticoagulants (blood thinners), ask your doctor before starting a cure!!!
- Do not use if you are allergic to any ingredient
- Contact your doctor with any questions or concerns

Disclaimer: This does not replace medical advice. Check With Your Doctor for symptoms or worsening of condition.

Amenorrhea

Amenorrhea is a condition characterized by the lack of menstruation in girls by the age 15 (primary amenorrhea) or in women by absence of 3 successive menstrual periods (secondary amenorrhea). Of course, pregnancy is the most common reason for amenorrhea, as well as breastfeeding.

Symptoms and signs:

- absence of menses
- pelvic pain
- milky nipple discharge
- headache
- acne and facial hair overgrowth

Seek medical advice for this condition, often there are reproductive organs problems or hormonal disturbances in the background.

Risk factors:

- stress
- eating disturbances such as bulimia, anorexia etc. and low body weight
- excessive physical activity
- relatives who suffered/suffer of this condition
- drugs: hormonal contraceptives, opiates (by long term use), anti-psychotics

Recipe 75 - Honey and Common Yarrow

Difficulty: +; Time: 30 minutes;

Ingredients:

- 1 1/2 teaspoon honey
- 1 teaspoon dried common yarrow
- 250 ml water

Preparation: Put 1 teaspoon dried common yarrow in 250 ml boiling water, let it infuse for 10 minutes, then filter it. After cooling, mix with honey.

How to take it: 1 cup twice a day, before meals.

Tips:

- Yarrow properties: contains vitamin C, minerals (calcium, chromium, cobalt, aluminium), flavonoids (tannins), coumarins, phytosterols (natural hormones), essential oils such as limonene, cineole, isoartemisia ketone, borneol, sabinene, terpineol, camphor, camphene, alpha and beta pinene, lactones (achillein, achilleic acid), etc.; anti-inflammatory, anti-microbial, antihelmintic, boosts immunity, decongestant, expectorant, pre-

vents gall stone formation, helps repairing the digestive tract lining, choleretic, cholagogue, diuretic, hemostatic, antispastic, regulates menstruation (hormonal regulator), skin conditions (eczema, wounds, burns).
- Yarrow beneficial effects: menstruation disturbances, chronic inflammation of ovaries, respiratory infections, stimulates digestion, prevents gall stones formation, abdominal cramps, enteritis, enterocolitis, diarrhea, billiary dyskinesia, hemorrhoids, skin wounds and burns (antiseptic, haemostatic, promotes healing), eczema.
- Use organic raw honey and yarrow.
- Use regularly for 7 days for better effects

Precautions:

- Yarrow contraindications: can cause contact allergies. May cause light sensitivity in predisposed persons. Avoid in pregnancy and breastfeeding. In high dose, it may cause dizziness and headaches.
- Do not use if you are allergic to any ingredient
- Contact your doctor with any questions or concerns

Disclaimer: This does not replace medical advice. Check With Your Doctor for symptoms or worsening of condition.

Recipe 76 - Honey and Caraway

Difficulty: +; Time: 2-3 minutes;

Ingredients:
- 1 tablespoon honey
- 1 teaspoon caraway seeds (actual fruits)

Preparation: Mix honey with caraway fruits.

How to take it: In the morning and in the evening, 30 minutes before meals.

Tips:
- Caraway properties: vitamins (A, B complex, C, E), minerals (calcium, magnesium, zinc, iron, copper, manganese), flavonoids (lutein, beta-carotene, cryptoxanthin), volatile oils (carveol, fufurol, carvone, etc.); lowers cholesterol, anti-oxidant, anti-inflammatory, antiseptic, helps with cough, anti-flatulent, boosts immunity, stimulates and balances the female hormonal activity, triggers menstruation, diminishes pre-menstrual syndrome, stimulates lactate production, vermifuge.
- Caraway beneficial effects: high blood pressure, respiratory and other infections, arthritis,

rheumatism, gout, dyspepsia, irritable bowel syndrome, antihelmintic (intestinal worms), reduced milk secretion, pre-menstrual syndrome, dysmenorrhea (irregular and painful menstruation).
- Use organic raw honey and caraway.
- Use regularly for better effects

Precautions:

- Caraway seeds contraindications: high doses may affect kidneys and liver.
- Do not use if you are allergic to any ingredient
- Contact your doctor with any questions or concerns

Disclaimer: This does not replace medical advice. Check With Your Doctor for symptoms or worsening of condition.

Dysmenorrhea (Menstrual cramps)

Dysmenorrhea is a condition in which menstruation is accompanied by cramping pains. In some women, it may be severe enough to intrude in the daily activities.

Symptoms:

- pain (cramping or dull ache) in the lower abdomen or pelvis, that may radiate to the thighs and lower back
- nausea
- headache
- loose stools

Seek medical advice if the condition interferes with normal life, if there is a worsening of it, or a sudden severe onset, as the underlying cause may be a treatable disease (uterine fibroids, endometriosis)

Risk factors:

- smoking
- relatives with the condition
- irregular or abundant bleeding

Recipe 77 - Honey and Corn Silk

Difficulty: +; Time: 5 minutes;

Ingredients:

- 1 teaspoon honey
- 1 teaspoon corn silk powder

Preparation: Mix honey with corn silk powder.

How to take it: Take the mixture 3 times a day, 30 minutes before meals.

Tips:

- Corn silk properties: contains vitamins (A, B complex, C, E), minerals (magnesium, iron, zinc, potassium, phosphorous), betaine, flavonoids (tannins), alantoine, volatile oils, ergosterine, proteins (zeine, with high content of leucine and glutamic acid), starch; antispastic, diuretic, haemostatic, improves liver function, anti-inflammatory, astringent; in high doses, decreases blood sugar.
- Corn silk beneficial effects: kidney stones, urinary tract infections, prostatitis, cardio-vascular conditions, arthritis, rheumatism, high blood pressure, dysmenorrhea, menopause, edema, ascitis, helps with weight-loss.

- Use organic raw honey and corn silk.
- Use in cures of 4 weeks, then 1 week pause, for better effects

Precautions:

- Corn silk: avoid in pregnancy, precaution in diabetes, hypertension (interaction with Captopril, Enalapril, Furosemid), simultaneous administration of anti-inflammatory drugs which lower blood potassium; can reduce the efficacy of warfarin. Seek medical advice before starting the treatment.
- Do not use if you are allergic to any ingredient
- Contact your doctor with any questions or concerns

Disclaimer: This does not replace medical advice. Check With Your Doctor for symptoms or worsening of condition.

Recipe 78 - Honey and Dill

Difficulty: +; Time: 15 minutes;

Ingredients:
- 2 tablespoons honey
- 3 teaspoons dried dill
- 750 ml water

Preparation: Infuse 3 teaspoons of dried dill in 750 ml boiling water for 10 minutes, let it cool, then mix with honey. Store in the fridge.

How to take it: 1 cup 3 times a day, 30 minutes before meals.

Tips:

- Dill properties: contains vitamins (A, B complex, C), minerals (potassium, calcium, magnesium, phosphorous, manganese), flavonoids (beta-carotene equivalents); anti-inflammatory, diuretic, antispastic, lowers cholesterol, estrogenic, stimulates and balances the female hormonal activity, triggers menstruation, stimulates lactate production.
- Dill beneficial effects: high blood pressure, adjuvant in amenorrhea, reduced milk secretion,

dysmenorrhea (irregular and painful mentruation), female sterility, premature menopause, mammary hypoplasia (small breasts), dyspepsia, flatulence (fermentation colitis), gall bladder dyskinesia, urinary infections, helps with weight-loss.
- Use organic raw honey and dill seeds.
- Use regularly for better effects

Precautions:

- Dill contraindications: pregnancy, hyperestrogenism, hypermenorrhea, ovarian cysts, mammary nodules, mammary and genital tumors.
- Do not use if you are allergic to any ingredient
- Contact your doctor with any questions or concerns

Disclaimer: This does not replace medical advice. Check With Your Doctor for symptoms or worsening of condition.

Hypocalcaemia

Hypocalcaemia is a condition which includes a group of signs and symptoms resulting from disturbances in electricity conduction in the body, affecting the function of the nervous system and muscles, and the bone integrity. Objectively, there is a low blood level of calcium. In most cases, the underlying problem is either a vitamin D, or a magnesium deficiency.

Symptoms and signs:

- tingling or sensation of pins and needles (paresthesia) in limbs and around the mouth
- muscle spasms and stiffness, problems with speaking and swallowing
- fatigue
- irritability, anxiety, and even depression
- long-term hypocalcaemia leads to dry skin, eczema, brittle nails, cataracts, dementia, calcium deposits in the body (such as kidney stones), etc.

Severe symptoms:

- tetany: carpopedal (strong, persistent contractions of the hands and feet) and generalized (sustained, intense contractions in large muscles of the body); laryngospasms; seizures; palpitations

Seek medical advice!!!

Risk factors:

- lifestyle: insufficient dietary intake of calcium, magnesium and vitamin D, decreased sun exposure, stress and anxiety, intense physical exercise
- eating disorders, gastrointestinal disorders (prolonged vomiting, intestinal malabsorption, diarrhea, constipation, pancreatitis, liver failure), long-term use of magnesium-containing laxatives, kidney failure
- drugs: anticonvulsants (Phenobarbital, Phenytoin), Rifampin, etc.

Recipe 79 - Honey and Chicken Egg Shells

Difficulty: ++; Time: 7 days;

Ingredients:

- 6 tablespoons honey
- Shells from 20 large chicken eggs

Preparation: Gather the shells from 20 chicken eggs. Wash them thoroughly (do not remove the inside membrane), boil them for 5 minutes, let them dry, then crush them into powder. Mix honey with the eggshell powder, and let them macerate in a dark glass jar for 1 week.

How to take it: 1 tablespoon, in the morning, 30 minutes before meal.

Tips:

- Egg shell properties: calcium, magnesium, phophorous, sodium, potassium, iron, zinc, sulphur, silicon, aluminum, gelatin, collagen, amino acids (methionine, lysine, cisteine, isoleucine).
- Egg shell beneficial effects: excellent calcium source, in hypoparathyroidismus, osteoporosis, osteoarthritis, for teeth, paradontosis, pregnancy, difficult healing of fractures.

HONEY – THE NATURE'S GOLD RECIPES FOR HEALTH

- Use organic raw honey and eggs.
- Use in 3-week cure, then pause 2 weeks.

Precautions:

- Do not use if you are allergic to any ingredient
- Contact your doctor with any questions or concerns

Disclaimer: This does not replace medical advice. Check With Your Doctor for symptoms or worsening of condition.

Recipe 80 - Honey, Chicken Egg Shells and White Wine

Difficulty: ++; Time: 7 days;

Ingredients:

- 400 g honey
- Shells from 20 large chicken eggs
- 200 ml white wine

Preparation: Gather the shells from 20 chicken eggs. Wash them thoroughly (do not remove the inside membrane), boil them for 5 minutes, let them dry, then crush them into powder. Mix honey and white wine with the eggshell powder, and let them macerate in a dark glass jar for 1 week, stirring 3-4 times daily.

How to take it: 1 tablespoon 3 times a day (mixed in a glass with water), 30 minutes before meals. In children, only 1 teaspoon in the morning and at lunch time, 30 minutes before meals. In elderly persons, use only half of the adult dose.

Tips:

- Egg shell properties: calcium, magnesium, phophorous, sodium, potassium, iron, zinc, sulphur, silicon, aluminum, gelatin, collagen, amino acids (methionine, lysine, cisteine, isoleucine).
- Egg shell beneficial effects: excellent calcium source, in hypoparathyroidismus, osteoporosis, osteoarthritis, for teeth, paradontosis, pregnancy, difficult healing of fractures.
- Use organic raw honey and eggs.
- Use in 3-week cure, then pause 2 weeks.

Precautions:

- Do not use if you are allergic to any ingredient
- Contact your doctor with any questions or concerns

Disclaimer: This does not replace medical advice. Check With Your Doctor for symptoms or worsening of condition.

Osteoporosis

Osteoporosis is a condition characterized by low bone mass, consequence of lower bone production than the normal bone-loss. The higher bone weakness leads to fractures following falls or just mild stresses (such as coughing). Most commonly, the fractures occur in the spine, hip and wrist. Osteoporosis symptomatic is actually the symptomatic of osteoporotic fractures.

Symptoms and signs:

- back pain (collapsed or fractured vertebra)
- fractures occurring due to minor stresses
- over time a stooped posture and loss of height

Risk factors:

- lifestyle: lack of physical activity, dietary factors (insufficient calcium intake, eating disorders with extremely reduced food intake, stomach and intestine reducing surgery, soft drinks consumption), chronic alcohol and tobacco abuse.

- older women of white or Asian descendence, relatives with osteoporosis diseases: hormonal disturbances (lower than normal sex hormone levels, over-active thyroid, parathyroids and adrenal glands), inflammatory bowel disease, celiac disease, liver disturbances, kidney disease, cancer, rheumatoid arthritis, lupus.
- drugs: steroids (cortisone, prednisone), L-Thyroxine, anticonvulsants (phenytoin, barbiturates), anticoagulants (heparin, warfarin), aromatase inhibitors, thiazolidinediones (pioglitazone, rosiglitazone), proton pump inhibitors (omeprazole, lansoprazole), lithium.

Recipe 81 - Honey, Garlic and Apple Cider Vinegar

Difficulty: +; Time: 5- minute preparation; 1 week maceration;

Ingredients:

- 300 g honey
- 8 garlic cloves
- 300 ml apple cider vinegar

Preparation: Mix honey with crushed cloves to make a paste, then add apple cider vinegar and stir well. Store in the fridge for 7 days; stir it daily.

How to take it: 1 tablespoon mixed with 1 glass water, in the morning before breakfast.

Tips:

- Garlic properties: contains vitamins (A, B complex, C, K), minerals (calcium, magnesium, iron, manganese, potassium, selenium, zinc, phosphorous), thiosulfinates (allicin, methyl allyl sulfinates), ajoenes, sulfides, sulfoxides (alliin, isoalliin, methiin, garlicins), flavonoids (beta-carotene, lutein, zeaxanthin); anti-bacterial, anti-viral, anti-fungal, anti-inflammatory, anti-oxidant, anti-

platelet activity, decreases cholesterol, lowers blood sugar, lowers blood pressure.
• Garlic beneficial effects: heart diseases, high blood pressure, osteoporosis, various cancers, respiratory infections, sinusitis, asthma, gastric and duodenal ulcers, especially associated with *Helicobacter pylori*, liver cirrhosis, improves performance and reduces fatigue, detoxifies the body of heavy metals.
• Apple cider vinegar properties: contains vitamins (B complex, C, pantothenic acid), minerals (calcium, potassium, sodium, iron, phosphorus), acetic acid, malic acid, pectin, polyphenols (flavonols, flavanols, tannins, anthocyanins, dihydrochalcones, hidroxycinnamic acids); boosts immunity, anti-microbial, anti-inflammatory, antioxidant, lowers cholesterol, lowers blood sugar, acts as anti-acid.
• Apple cider vinegar beneficial effects: in infections (sinusitis, sore throat, asthma, other respiratory infections, urinary tract infections, etc), allergies, arthritis, gout, cardiovascular diseases, improves digestion, prevents constipation, helps with weight loss, in skin conditions (acne, eczema).
• Use organic raw honey, garlic and apple cider vinegar.
• Use regularly for better effects

Precautions:

• Garlic: may lower Saquinavir levels and may interact with some anticoagulants and diabetes medication. If you are on anticoagulants (blood

thinners), ask your doctor before starting a cure!!! May cause flatulence and nausea. Locally applied may lead to irritation, urticaria, anaphylaxis.
- Do not use if you are allergic to any ingredient
- Contact your doctor with any questions or concerns

Disclaimer: This does not replace medical advice. Check With Your Doctor for symptoms or worsening of condition.

Recipe 82 - Honey, Chicken Egg Shells and Lemon

Difficulty: ++; Time: 7 days;

Ingredients:

- 400 g honey
- Shells from 20 large chicken eggs
- 150 ml lemon juice

Preparation: Gather the shells from 20 chicken eggs. Wash them thoroughly (do not remove the inside membrane), boil them for 5 minutes, let them dry, then crush them into powder. Mix honey and lemon juice with the eggshell powder, and let them macerate in a dark glass jar for 1 week, stirring 3-4 times daily.

How to take it: 1 tablespoon 3 times a day (mixed in a glass with water), 30 minutes before meals. In children, only 1 teaspoon in the morning and at lunch time, 30 minutes before meals. In elderly persons, use only half of the adult dose.

Tips:

- Egg shell properties: calcium, magnesium, phophorous, sodium, potassium, iron, zinc, sulphur, silicon, aluminum, gelatin, collagen, amino acids (methionine, lysine, cisteine, isoleucine).
- Egg shell beneficial effects: excellent calcium source, in hypoparathyroidismus, osteoporosis, osteoarthritis, for teeth, paradontosis, pregnancy, difficult healing of fractures.
- Lemon properties: contains vitamins (A, B complex, C, E), minerals (calcium, magnesium, potassium, copper, manganese, zinc, iron), flavonoids (naringin, naringenin, hesperetin, alfa- and beta-carotenes, lutein, zeaxanthin, beta-cryptoxanthin, tannins), terpenes, citric acid, fibers; anti-oxidant, anti-inflammatory, anti-bacterial, antifungal, antiseptic, immune system booster.
- Lemon beneficial effects: dyspepsia, constipation, respiratory infections, asthma, rheumatism, arthritis, lowers blood pressure, helps with weight-loss, anti-cancer, acne, eczema, burns.
- Use organic raw honey, lemon and eggs.
- Use in 3-week cure, then pause 2 weeks.

Precautions:

- Lemon may cause photosensitivity when used on skin.
- Do not use if you are allergic to any ingredient
- Contact your doctor with any questions or concerns

Disclaimer: This does not replace medical advice. Check With Your Doctor for symptoms or worsening of condition.

Chapter 9

Nervous System Diseases

Anxiety

Anxiety includes a group of disorders with the core trait an excessive, continuous fear and worry regarding everyday events. It involves frequently bouts of intense anxiety or terror: panic attacks, which impede normal daily activities.

Such disorders are specific phobias (agoraphobia, claustrophobia, etc.), generalized anxiety disorder, stranger anxiety, etc. They may be associated with or a consequence of another medical disorder.

Symptoms and signs:

- having feelings of restlessness and nervousness, and the sensation of panic or imminent danger
- trembling and sweating
- feeling exhausted
- fast breathing and accelerated heart rate
- insomnia

- having trouble to control worry, to focus on other things
- compulsively evading the anxiety triggers

Seek medical advice if worrying impacts your life, if feeling depressed, having suicidal ideas, or suspecting an underlying disease.

Risk factors:

- stress
- drugs, alcohol
- other mental health conditions
- after traumatic events
- relatives with anxiety

Recipe 83 - Honey and Hawthorn (macerate)

Difficulty: +; Time: 1 month;

Ingredients:
- 1 kg honey
- 700 g fresh hawthorn fruits

Preparation: Mix honey with fresh hawthorn fruits and put the mixture in a sealed jar. Store it in a cool and dark place for a month. Filter the content, and pour the syrup in dark glass bottles.

How to take it: 1 teaspoon 3 times a day, 30 minutes before meals.

Tips:

- Hawthorn properties: contains vitamins (B, C, E), flavonoids (tannins, epicatechin, quercetin, rutin, C-glycosylated flavone derivative, hyperoside, kaempferol, anthocyanin, anthocyanidins), triterpenes, chlorogenic acids, organic acids (citric, nicotinic, malic), volatile oils; anti-oxidant, anti-inflammatory, sedativ, cardiotonic, cardioprotective, hypolipidaemic, antiarrhytmic, coronary vasodilator, lowers blood pressure.

- Hawthorn beneficial effects: anxiety, depression, migraines, insomnia, high blood pressure, ischemic cardiomyopathie, cardiac insufficiency, palpitations.
- Use organic raw honey and hawthorn.
- Use regularly for better effects

Precautions:

- Hawthorn: avoid in pregnancy. In high dose, may reduce blood pressure and cause dizziness and faint. May increase the activity of digoxine, beta-blockers, calcium channel blockers, and anti-depressives. If you are on anticoagulants (blood thinners), ask your doctor before starting a cure!!!
- Do not use if you are allergic to any ingredient
- Contact your doctor with any questions or concerns

Disclaimer: This does not replace medical advice. Check With Your Doctor for symptoms or worsening of condition.

Recipe 84 - Honey and Celery Juice

Difficulty: +; Time: 5 minutes;

Ingredients:

- 1/2 tablespoon honey
- 250 ml celery juice

Preparation: Mix honey with celery juice.

How to take it: 1 glass 3 times a day, 30 minutes before meals.

Tips:

- Celery properties: contains vitamins (A, B complex, C), minerals (calcium, magnesium, potassium, sodium, iron, zinc, phosphorous, etc), flavonoids (beta-caroten, lutein, zeaxanthin, flavonols: quercetin, kampferol), essential oils (apiol, sedanolide), furanocoumarins (psoralen, bergapten), linoleic acid, lunularin, terpenes, 3-n-butyl-phtalide; anti-oxidant, anti-inflammatory, anti-microbial, stimulates digestion, diuretic, expectorant, lowers cholesterol, calming effect.
- Celery beneficial effects: kidney infections and stones, lowers high blood pressure, respiratory infections (asthma, bronchitis), helps with

stress, arthritis, rheumatism, gout, in mouth ulcers, gingivitis, helps with gastro-duodenal ulcers, liver detoxification, constipation, helps with weight-loss, diabetes, skin wounds.
- Use organic raw honey and celery.
- Use regularly for better effects

Precautions:

- Celery: may cause allergy and photosensibilisation. Avoid in pregnancy. If you are on anticoagulants (blood thinners), ask your doctor before starting a cure!!!
- Do not use if you are allergic to any ingredient
- Contact your doctor with any questions or concerns

Disclaimer: This does not replace medical advice. Check With Your Doctor for symptoms or worsening of condition.

Anorexia

Anorexia represents an eating disorder defined by very low body weight, a twisted notion regarding body weight and extreme fear about gaining weight. In order to control their weight, the persons affected by this disease severely restrict food intake, or use other "control" methods such as vomiting following meals, laxatives, enemas, or excessive physical exercise.

Symptoms and signs:

- exaggerated low body weight
- fatigue and insomnia
- thin hair that breaks
- dry, yellowish skin
- swelling of limbs
- absence of menstruation
- palpitations, low blood pressure
- exaggerated restriction of food intake, bingeing, use of laxatives, excessive preoccupation with weight gaining, lack of emotion or irritability, depression, suicide ideas.

Seek medical advice when experiencing the above-mentioned symptoms.

Risk factors:

- female gender, with male gender "catching up"
- transition periods or stressful events
- relatives with anorexia
- certain professions, such as those in artistic or sports related fields

Recipe 85 - Honey, Red Wine and Horseradish

Difficulty: ++; Time: 10 days;

Ingredients:
- 400 g honey
- 20 tablespoons grated horseradish
- 1 liter red wine

Preparation: Mix honey with grated horseradish and wine. Let it to macerate for 10 days, then filter it.

How to take it: 1 tablespoon 3 times a day, 30 minutes before meals.

Tips:

- Horseradish properties: contains vitamins (A, B complex, C - high content), minerals (calcium, magnesium, iron, phosphorous, zinc, copper, manganese), flavonoids (beta-carotene, lutein, zeaxanthin) glutamines, asparagine, sinigrin (a glucosinolate), allyl isothiocyanate; cardiotonic, anti-oxidant, anti-inflammatory, relaxant, expectorant, laxative.

- Horseradish beneficial effects: lowers blood pressure, helps in angina pectoris, respiratory infections, cold, sinusitis, bronchitis, asthma, helps in anorexia etc.
- Use organic raw honey, horseradish and wine.
- Use regularly for better effects

Precautions:

- Horseradish contraindications: palpitations (cardiac rhythm disturbances), hemorrhoids.
- Do not use if you are allergic to any ingredient
- Contact your doctor with any questions or concerns

Disclaimer: This does not replace medical advice. Check With Your Doctor for symptoms or worsening of condition.

Recipe 86 - Honey and Dates

Difficulty: +; Time: 12 hours;

Ingredients:

- 3 teaspoons honey
- 4 - 5 dried dates

Preparation: Mix honey with the crushed dates and with 250 ml lukewarm water. Store in the fridge overnight.

How to take it: In the morning before breakfast.

Tips:

- Dates properties: contain vitamins (A, B complex, K), minerals (calcium, magnesium, potassium, sodium, iron, phosphorus, zinc, manganese), flavonoids (beta-carotene, cryptoxanthin, zeahanthin, luteine), phenolic acids, carbohydrates (high content), fibers; antioxidants, anti-microbial, anti-cancer, lower cholesterol, hepatoprotective, expectorant.
- Dates beneficial effects: in constipation, intestinal disorders, anemia, heart problems, sexual dysfunctions, osteoporosis, for gaining weight,

stimulate digestion, prevent heart disorders, in neuritis, pulmonary infections (bronchitis).
- Use organic raw honey and dates.
- Use regularly for better effects

Precautions:

- Dates contraindication: in diabetes mellitus (high sugar content).
- Do not use if you are allergic to any ingredient
- Contact your doctor with any questions or concerns

Disclaimer: This does not replace medical advice. Check With Your Doctor for symptoms or worsening of condition.

Alzheimer's Disease

Alzheimer's disease is a progressive chronic neurodegenerative condition, affecting memory and other mental functions. It is the most common cause of dementia.

Symptoms and signs:

- short-term memory loss or a mild confusion are the most often early symptoms
- disorientation, difficulty focusing and thinking
- troubles in organizing familiar tasks and making decisions
- progressive personality changes and mood swings, social withdrawal, changes in sleeping pattern, delusions, and other behavioral changes
- self-care, enjoying old music, reading, hobby practicing, storytelling, etc. remain unchanged until the late stages

Risk factors:

- life style - smoking, dietary habits, obesity, lack of physical exercise, lack of involvement in social and mental activities
- previous serious head trauma
- mild cognitive impairment
- relatives with Alzheimer's disease
- aging and female gender
- other diseases (cardiovascular, Down syndrome, uncontrolled type 2 diabetes mellitus)

Recipe 87 - Honey and European Blueberry

Difficulty: +; Time: 5 minutes; 8 hours to macerate;

Ingredients:

- 4 teaspoons honey
- 4 teaspoons powdered blueberries
- 500 ml water

Preparation: Mix powdered berries with warm water (not more than 40°C). Let it macerate for 8 hours, then mix with honey.

How to take it: 1/2 of the quantity, twice a day, in the morning before breakfast and at bed time.

Tips:

- Blueberry properties: contains vitamins (A, B, C, E, F, PP), minerals (calcium, magnesium, iron, manganese, selenium, zinc), flavonoids (anthocyanins, quercetin, catechins, tannins, ellagitannins), aleagic acid, fibers; anti-oxidant, anti-inflammatory, antibacterial, boosts immunity, anti-cancer, lowers cholesterol and triglycerides, cardioprotective, lowers blood pressure, antithrombotic, neuroprotective.

- Blueberry beneficial effects: cardio-vascular conditions, varicose veins, respiratory and urinary infections, neuro-degenerative disorders (Alzheimer, vascular dementia), chronic fatigue, obesity, anti-cancer, rheumatoid arthritis, gout.
- Use organic raw honey and blueberries.
- For better effects, do not filter. A cure lasts 2 weeks to 1 month.

Precautions:

- Blueberry contraindications: gastric ulcer, gastritis, gall bladder inflammation.
- Do not use if you are allergic to any ingredient
- Contact your doctor with any questions or concerns

Disclaimer: This does not replace medical advice. Check With Your Doctor for symptoms or worsening of condition.

Recipe 88 - Honey, Onion Juice and Black Pepper

Difficulty: +; Time: 2-3 minutes;

Ingredients:

- 1 tablespoon honey
- 1 pinch black pepper
- juice from 1 medium onion
- 1 glass water

Preparation: Mix honey with water, onion juice and pepper.

How to take it: In the morning before breakfast.

Tips:

- Black pepper properties: contains vitamins (A, B complex, C, E, K), choline, minerals (calcium, magnesium, manganese, copper, iron, zinc), piperine (essential oil), monoterpenes (pinene, sabinene, mercene, limonene, terpenene), flavonoids (carotenes, lycopene, zea-xanthin, cryptoxanthin); antioxidant, anti-inflammatory, anti-bacterial, analgesic, carminative, anti-flatulent.
- Black pepper beneficial effects: respiratory infections, asthma, weight loss, constipation, ane-

mia, gastric and duodenal ulcers, ear- and toothaches, heart disease, cognitive impairment (Alzheimer's disease, dementia), and helps with vitiligo.
- Onion properties: contains vitamins (B complex, C, D), minerals (calcium, magnesium, potassium, copper, phosphorus, manganese), flavonoids (quercetin, fisetin, tannins, anthocyanins), thiosulfinates, fiber; anti-oxidant, anti-inflammatory, decreases cholesterol, improves mood and lowers blood sugar, anti-cancer.
- Onion beneficial effects: prevention and improvement in heart diseases, respiratory infections, asthma, sinusitis, depression, improves sleep.
- Use organic raw honey, onion and black pepper.
- Use regularly for better effects

Precautions:

- Black pepper may cause skin irritation after direct application; consumed in large amounts in pregnancy may induce miscarriage, and high intake is not recommended in ulcers.
- Onion may cause bloating, in high amounts may interfere with blood thinning. If you are on anticoagulants (blood thinners), ask your doctor before starting a cure!!!
- Do not use if you are allergic to any ingredient
- Contact your doctor with any questions or concerns

Disclaimer: This does not replace medical advice. Check With Your Doctor for symptoms or worsening of condition.

Recipe 89 - Honey and Orange Juice

Difficulty: +; Time: 2-3 minutes;

Ingredients:

- 1 tablespoon honey
- 1 glass of orange juice

Preparation: Mix honey with juice.

How to take it: In the morning before breakfast.

Tips:

- Orange properties: contains vitamins (A, B complex, C, D, E), calcium, magnesium, phosphorous, zinc, copper, potassium, flavonoids (naringenin, hesperetin, alpha- and beta-carotens, lutein, zeaxanthin), limonoids (limonin glucosyde), pectin, fats, fibers; anti-oxidant, boosts immunity, lowers blood pressure, lowers cholesterol and triglycerides, decreases insulin resistance, anti-cancer.
- Orange beneficial effects: infections, degenerative diseases (Alzheimer's disease, Parkinson disease), fatigue, cardio-vascular diseases, prevents kidney stones, helps with digestion, constipation, flatulence, helps with weight-loss.

- Use organic raw honey and orange.
- Use regularly for better effects

Precautions:

- Do not use if you are allergic to any ingredient
- Contact your doctor with any questions or concerns

Disclaimer: This does not replace medical advice. Check With Your Doctor for symptoms or worsening of condition.

Recipe 5 - Honey and Turmeric

Recipe 118 - Honey and Common Sea Buckthorn

Depression

Depression is a condition in which the mood is affected, causing a continuous feeling of sadness and a disinterest in general, which results in a disruption of the daily activities and sometimes even in the occurrence of suicidal thoughts.

Symptoms:

- episodes of sadness, hopelessness or tearfulness along with explosions of irritability and angriness
- disinterest in normal activities and feelings of worthlessness
- restlessness, agitation, insomnia or oversleeping, lack of appetite or overeating
- fatigue, slow thinking, focusing, and slow body movements
- repeated suicidal thoughts or suicide

Seek medical advice if experiencing the above-mentioned symptoms.

Risk factors:

- stressful events
- other mental health disturbances
- chronic alcoholism or recreational drugs consumption
- relatives with depression or other mental health disorders
- drugs, such as sleeping pills

Recipe 90 - Honey and Common Sea Buckthorn

Difficulty: +; Time: 30 minutes;

Ingredients:

- 500 g honey
- 700 g fresh sea buckthorn fruits

Preparation: Mix crushed sea buckthorn fruits with honey in a jar. Seal it tightly and let the content to macerate for 10 days. Store in the fridge.

How to take it: 1 tablespoon in the morning, 30 minutes before meal.

Tips:

- Sea buckthorn properties: contains vitamins (A, B complex, C - high content, E, F, K, P), minerals (magnesium, calcium, phosphorus), flavonoids (quercetin, kaempherol, isorhamnetin, alpha- and beta-carotenoids, lutein, zeaxanthin, lycopene, catechins, epigallocatechins, gallocatechins), phytosterols, omega-3, omega-6, omega-7, omega-9 fatty acids, essential amino acids, tannins etc.; antioxidant, anti-inflammatory, stimulates immunity and wound healing.

- Sea buckthorn beneficial effects: infections (especially respiratory), digestive tract disorders (gastric ulcer, hepatitis), high blood pressure, coronary disease, eye disorders, skin conditions (eczema, psoriasis, dermatitis), rheumatism, neurologic disorders (asthenia, depression, Parkinson, Alzheimer).
- Use organic raw honey and sea buckthorn.
- Use regularly for a month. After 1-2 weeks pause, repeat the cure.

Precautions:

- Sea buckthorn contraindications: in inflammation of the gall bladder (acute cholecystitis) and pancreas (pancreatitis). It may lead to mastopathy in women and to adenomatous prostatitis (high content in phytohormones) in men, and in high amounts as well to allergie (in asthma and in rarely cases due to high quantities of beta-caroten).
- Do not use if you are allergic to any ingredient
- Contact your doctor with any questions or concerns

Disclaimer: This does not replace medical advice. Check With Your Doctor for symptoms or worsening of condition.

Recipe 91 - Honey and Onion

Difficulty: +; Time: 2-3 minutes;

Ingredients:
- 1 teaspoon honey
- 1 teaspoon onion juice

Preparation: Mix honey with the onion juice.

How to take it: 3 times a day, 30 minutes before meals.

Tips:
- Onion properties: contains vitamins (B complex, C, D), minerals (calcium, magnesium, potassium, copper, phosphorus, manganese), flavonoids (quercetin, fisetin, tannins, anthocyanins), thiosulfinates, fiber; anti-oxidant, anti-inflammatory, decreases cholesterol, improves mood and lowers blood sugar, anti-cancer.
- Onion beneficial effects: prevention and improvement in heart diseases, respiratory infections, asthma, sinusitis, depression, improves sleep.
- Use organic raw honey and onions.
- Use regularly for better effects.

Precautions:

- Onion may cause bloating, in high amounts may interfere with blood thinning. If you are on anticoagulants (blood thinners), ask your doctor before starting a cure!!!
- Do not use if you are allergic to any ingredient
- Contact your doctor with any questions or concerns

Disclaimer: This does not replace medical advice. Check With Your Doctor for symptoms or worsening of condition.

Recipe 5 - Honey and Turmeric

Chronic Fatigue Syndrome

Chronic fatigue syndrome is a condition characterized by severe fatigue, which doesn't ameliorate with rest. This overtiredness cannot be clarified by any underlying disease.

Symptoms and signs:

- severe fatigue over at least six months in a row
- over 24-hour serious exhaustion following mental or physical exercise
- unrefreshing sleep
- lack of concentration and impaired memory
- headaches of a new pattern or with increased severity
- muscle pain of unexplained cause
- often sore throat
- swollen and sore lymph nodes in the neck or armpits
- migratory pain in the joints without swelling, increased local temperature or redness
- brain fog, mood problems (depression, anxiety, etc.)
- constipation, diarrhea, nausea

Seek medical advice for extreme, unrelenting fatigue

Risk factors:

- stress
- age: more common around 40-50 years of age
- relatives with chronic fatigue syndrome
- preexistent mental health conditions (anxiety, depression)

Recipe 92 - Honey, Green Walnuts and Dog Rose

Difficulty: +; Time: 15 minutes;

Ingredients:
- 1 tablespoon honey
- 5 green walnuts
- 200 ml dog rose juice

Preparation: Mix honey with crushed green walnuts and make a paste. Dissolve the paste in the dog rose juice.

How to take it: In the morning, 30 minutes before meal.

Tips:
- Walnuts properties: vitamins (A, B complex, E), minerals (magnesium, zinc, manganese, molybdenum, copper, iron), flavonoids (beta-carotene, lutein, zeaxanthin), proteins (contain L-arginine, which is an essential amino acid); anti-oxidant, anti-inflammatory, lower cholesterol, increase insulin production, laxative.
- Walnuts beneficial effects: prevention of cardio-vascular diseases, lower blood pressure, prevent macular degeneration and cataract,

asthma, rheumatoid arthritis, psoriasis, eczema, improve depression, prevent gallstones, constipation, Type 2 diabetes, great for hair and skin.
- Dog rose properties: contains vitamins (A, B complex, C - high amounts, E, F), minerals (magnesium, calcium, manganese, selenium, iron, zinc, phosphorous, sulfur), flavonoids (carotenoids, tannins), terpenoids, organic acids; reduces small blood vessels fragility, anti-oxidant, anti-inflammatory, lowers blood sugar, boosts immunity, promotes regeneration, diuretic, stimulates uric acid removal.
- Dog rose beneficial effects: improves peripheral circulation, reduces atherosclerosis, respiratory and urinary infections, rheumatism, gout, gall bladder disorders, kidney diseases, general tonic.
- Use organic raw honey, walnuts and dog rose juice.
- Use regularly for 1 month for better effects

Precautions:

- Walnuts: may trigger allergy, even anaphylaxis; when used on skin may cause rash; may cause loose stools.
- Dog rose contraindications: avoid use during pregnancy or lactation.
- Do not use if you are allergic to any ingredient
- Contact your doctor with any questions or concerns

HONEY – THE NATURE'S GOLD RECIPES FOR HEALTH

Disclaimer: This does not replace medical advice. Check With Your Doctor for symptoms or worsening of condition.

Recipe 93 - Honey, Green Walnuts and Cloves

Difficulty: ++; Time: 45 minutes;

Ingredients:
- 750 g honey
- 20 green walnuts
- 10 cloves
- 1 liter water

Preparation: Boil finely chopped green walnuts peels for 10 minutes in 1 liter water, then add the cloves and let it cool. Filter the mixture, add the honey and stir well. Store it in the fridge in dark bottles.

How to take it: 1 teaspoon 3 times a day, 30 minutes before meals.

Tips:

- Walnuts properties: vitamins (A, B complex, E), minerals (magnesium, zinc, manganese, molybdenum, copper, iron), flavonoids (beta-carotene, lutein, zeaxanthin), proteins (contain L-arginine, which is an essential amino acid); anti-oxidant, anti-inflammatory, lower cholesterol, increase insulin production, laxative.

- Walnuts beneficial effects: prevention of cardio-vascular diseases, lower blood pressure, prevent macular degeneration and cataract, asthma, rheumatoid arthritis, psoriasis, eczema, improve depression, prevent gallstones, constipation, Type 2 diabetes, great for hair and skin.
- Cloves properties: contain vitamins (A, B complex, C, K), minerals (calcium, magnesium, copper, iron, manganese, selenium, zinc, phosphorous), flavonoids (rhamnetin, eugenin, eugenitin, kaempferol, beta-carotene, tannins such as methyl salicylate, gallotannic acid), essential oils (acetyl eugenol, vanillin, maslinic acid, β-caryophyllene), triterpenoids (campesterol, stigmasterol, oleanolic acid); anti-oxidant, anti-inflammatory, antiseptic, anti-bacterial, fight against intestinal parasites, analgesic, boost the immune system, lower blood sugar, anti-nausea, dyspepsia, anti-flatulent, reduce stress, anti-cancer.
- Cloves beneficial effects: asthma, respiratory infections, sinusitis, rheumatism, gout, improve digestion, acne, diabetes.
- Use organic raw honey, green walnuts and cloves.
- Use regularly for better effects

Precautions:

- Walnuts: may trigger allergy, even anaphylaxis; when used on skin may cause rash; may cause loose stools.
- Cloves contraindications: avoid in pregnancy, stomach ulcers or if under treatment with anticoagulants. If you are on anticoagulants (blood thinners), ask your doctor before starting a cure!!!
- Do not use if you are allergic to any ingredient
- Contact your doctor with any questions or concerns

Disclaimer: This does not replace medical advice. Check With Your Doctor for symptoms or worsening of condition.

Recipe 94 - Honey, Carrots and Celery Juice

Difficulty: +; Time: 5 minutes;

Ingredients:

- 1/2 tablespoon honey
- 100 ml carrot juice
- 100 ml celery juice

Preparation: Mix honey with the carrot and celery juice.

How to take it: 1 glass 3 times a day, 30 minutes before meals.

Tips:

- Carrot properties: contains vitamins (A, B complex, C, E, K), minerals (copper, manganese, molybdenum), carotenoids (alfa- and beta-caroten, lutein), anthocyanindins, hydroxycinamic acid, high fiber content; anti-oxidant, anti-inflammatory, antibacterial, detoxifying, lowers cholesterol, lowers insulin resistance, boosts immunity.
- Carrot beneficial effects: prevents macular degeneration, improves vision, prevents heart disease, stroke, helps with gum and teeth disorders, improves digestion, anti-cancer.

- Celery properties: contains vitamins (A, B complex, C), minerals (calcium, magnesium, potassium, sodium, iron, zinc, phosphorous, etc), flavonoids (beta-caroten, lutein, zeaxanthin, flavonols: quercetin, kampferol), essential oils (apiol, sedanolide), furanocoumarins (psoralen, bergapten), linoleic acid, lunularin, terpenes, 3-n-butyl-phtalide; anti-oxidant, anti-inflammatory, anti-microbial, stimulates digestion, diuretic, expectorant, lowers cholesterol, calming effect.
- Celery beneficial effects: kidney infections and stones, lowers high blood pressure, respiratory infections (asthma, bronchitis), helps with stress, arthritis, rheumatism, gout, in mouth ulcers, gingivitis, helps with gastro-duodenal ulcers, liver detoxification, constipation, helps with weight-loss, diabetes, skin wounds.
- Use organic raw honey, carrots and celery.
- Use regularly for better effects

Precautions:

- Consumed in excess, carrots may color the skin orange (face, palms, feet). Avoid in small intestine inflammation, acute gastro-duodenal ulcer.
- Celery: may cause allergy and photosensibilisation. Avoid in pregnancy. If you are on anticoagulants (blood thinners), ask your doctor before starting a cure!!!
- Do not use if you are allergic to any ingredient
- Contact your doctor with any questions or concerns

Disclaimer: This does not replace medical advice. Check With Your Doctor for symptoms or worsening of condition.

Recipe 95 - Honey and Liquorice (decoction)

Difficulty: +; Time: 30 minutes;

Ingredients:

- 1 tablespoon honey
- 1 1/2 teaspoons powder liquorice
- 250 ml water

Preparation: Boil 1 1/2 teaspoons powdered liquorice in 250 ml hot water for 20 minutes, then let it cool and filter it. Mix the solution with the honey and stir thoroughly.

How to take it: 1 cup twice a day, 30 minutes before meals, not longer than 1 month.

Tips:

- Liquorice properties: contains vitamins (B complex, E), minerals (calcium, magnesium, phosphorous, silicon, iron, zinc, selenium), flavonoids (beta-carotene, quercetin), phenol, glycyrrhizin, thymol, glabridin, phytoestrogens; anti-oxidant, anti-inflammatory, expectorant, growth inhibition of *Helicobacter pylori*, anti-tumor, anti-microbial (also anti-Mycobacterial, antiviral), boosts immunity, lowers cholesterol.

- Liquorice beneficial effects: mouth aphtous ulcers, dyspepsia, gastric and duodenal ulcer associated with *Helicobacter pylori*, liver protection, rheumatism, gout, polyarthritis rheumatoides, menopause, pre-menstrual syndrome, chronic fatigue syndrome, pulmonary infections, pulmonary tuberculosis, acne, shingles, helps in HIV infection, prevention and treatment of cardio-vascular diseases.
- Use organic raw honey and liquorice.
- Use regularly for better effects

Precautions:

- Liquorice should not be administered during pregnancy, while under digitalis or steroids treatment or in case of renal dysfunction with impaired salt excretion. During the cure, a low salt diet is recommended. May cause body fatigue, kidney disorders, irregular menstruation, may interact with diuretics. Prolonged use may cause the retention of fluid in the body, high blood pressure, low blood potassium levels (hypokalemia), and cataracts.
- Do not use if you are allergic to any ingredient
- Contact your doctor with any questions or concerns

Disclaimer: This does not replace medical advice. Check With Your Doctor for symptoms or worsening of condition.

Chapter 10

Skin Diseases

Acne

Acne is a long-term, persistent skin condition characterized by the development of pimples, white or blackheads (comedones), as a result of hair follicles occlusion with dead skin cells as well as sebum (oil produced by the skin oil glands).

It occurs commonly on face, neck, shoulders, back and chest, where there is a higher number of oil glands. Acne is more frequent among teenagers. It can lead to scaring and, in severe cases, may associate with emotional damage ranging from low self esteem to depression.

Symptoms and signs:

- white or blackheads (comedones)
- pimples (pustules)
- painful, hard, sizable knots under the skin
- scars and pigmentation, reflecting an abnormal healing in untreated cases

Seek medical advice if persistent, severe symptomatology

Risk factors:

- stress - worsens the condition
- skin trauma (pressure, friction) caused by tight collars, chin straps, cell phones, backpacks etc.
- hormonal swings in teenagers, women, certain drugs used (corticoids, androgens, hydantoin, bromides, isoniazid, lithium, etc.)
- relatives suffering from acne
- a diet high in carbohydrates
- infections

Recipe 96 - Honey and Liquorice Powder

Difficulty: +; Time: 5 minutes;

Ingredients:

- 1 1/2 teaspoon honey
- 1 1/2 teaspoon liquorice powder

Preparation: Mix honey with liquorice powder.

How to take it: Apply mixture on the face or affected area. After 15 minutes, rinse it with warm water.

Tips:

- Liquorice properties: contains vitamins (B complex, E), minerals (calcium, magnesium, phosphorous, silicon, iron, zinc, selenium), flavonoids (beta-carotene, quercetin), phenol, glycyrrhizin, thymol, glabridin, phytoestrogens; anti-oxidant, anti-inflammatory, expectorant, growth inhibition of *Helicobacter pylori*, anti-tumor, anti-microbial (also anti-Mycobacterial, antiviral), boosts immunity, lowers cholesterol.
- Liquorice beneficial effects: mouth aphtous ulcers, dyspepsia, gastric and duodenal ulcer associated with *Helicobacter pylori*, liver protection,

rheumatism, gout, polyarthritis rheumatoides, menopause, pre-menstrual syndrome, chronic fatigue syndrome, pulmonary infections, pulmonary tuberculosis, acne, shingles, helps in HIV infection, prevention and treatment of cardio-vascular diseases.

- Use organic raw honey and liquorice.
- Use once per day for better effects

Precautions:

- Liquorice should not be administered during pregnancy, while under digitalis or steroids treatment or in case of renal dysfunction with impaired salt excretion. During the cure, a low salt diet is recommended. May cause body fatigue, kidney disorders, irregular menstruation, may interact with diuretics. Prolonged use may cause the retention of fluid in the body, high blood pressure, low blood potassium levels (hypokalemia), and cataracts. Use in 4 to 6-week cure, followed by 2 to 3-week pause.
- Do not use if you are allergic to any ingredient
- Contact your doctor with any questions or concerns

Disclaimer: This does not replace medical advice. Check With Your Doctor for symptoms or worsening of condition.

Recipe 97 - Honey and Potato

Difficulty: +; Time: 15 minutes;

Ingredients:

- 1 teaspoon honey
- 1 medium sized potato

Preparation: Mix honey with grated potato.

How to take it: Apply locally with a sterile gauze, for 2 hours, 2-3 times a day.

Tips:

- Potato properties: contains vitamins (B complex, C), minerals (calcium, potassium, magnesium, sodium, phosphorous, iron, manganese, copper), flavonoids (carotenes, zeaxanthins, quercetin) starch, fibers; emollient, anti-oxidant, analgesic, anti-inflammatory, heals wounds, antacid.
- Potato beneficial effects: conjunctivitis, tired eyes, cataracts, rheumatism, gout, skin lesions (acne, burns, eczema), hematomas, stomach and liver problems, lowers high blood pressure, depression, kidney stones, urinary tract infections.
- Use organic raw honey and potatoes.
- Use regularly for better effects

Precautions:

- Do not use if you are allergic to any ingredient
- Contact your doctor with any questions or concerns

Disclaimer: This does not replace medical advice. Check With Your Doctor for symptoms or worsening of condition.

Recipe 98 - Honey and Apple

Difficulty: +; Time: 10 minutes;

Ingredients:

- 1 1/2 tablespoon honey
- 1 medium apple

Preparation: Mix honey with grated apple.

How to take it: Apply mixture on the face or affected area. After 15 minutes, rinse it with warm water.

Tips:

- Apple properties: contains vitamins (A, B complex, C, E, PP), minerals (calcium, magnesium, iodine, iron, silicon, molybdenum, phosphorous), flavonoids (quercetin, kaempferol, myricetin, anthocyanins, epicatechin), chlorogenic acid, triterpenoids, fiber (high content); expectorant, anti-microbial, anti-oxidant, regulates cholesterol.
- Apple beneficial effects: infections, stress, depression, fatigue, colitis, billiary diskinesia, constipation, improves hemorrhoids, helps with weight-loss, rheumatism, gout, prevents cardio-

vascular disorders, wounds healing, burns, eczema, acne.
- Use organic raw honey and apples.
- Use regularly for better effects

Precautions:

- Do not use if you are allergic to any ingredient
- Contact your doctor with any questions or concerns

Disclaimer: This does not replace medical advice. Check With Your Doctor for symptoms or worsening of condition.

Recipe 99 - Honey, Yoghurt and Lemon

Difficulty: +; Time: 10 minutes;

Ingredients:

- 1 tablespoon honey
- 1 1/2 tablespoons yoghurt
- juice from 1/2 lemon

Preparation: Mix honey with yoghurt and lemon juice.

How to take it: Apply mixture on the face or affected area. After 15 minutes, rinse it with warm water.

Tips:

- Yoghurt properties: contains Lactobacillus acidophilus, vitamins (A, B complex, C, D), minerals (calcium, magnesium, potassium), proteins; probiotic, maintains a more acidic environment, lowers cholesterol, boosts immune system.
- Yoghurt beneficial effects: acne, vaginal infections, intestinal infections, flatulence, constipation, lactose intolerance, osteoporosis, hypertension.

- Lemon properties: contains vitamins (A, B complex, C, E), minerals (calcium, magnesium, potassium, copper, manganese, zinc, iron), flavonoids (naringin, naringenin, hesperetin, alfa- and beta-carotenes, lutein, zeaxanthin, beta-cryptoxanthin, tannins), terpenes, citric acid, fibers; anti-oxidant, anti-inflammatory, anti-bacterial, antifungal, antiseptic, immune system booster.
- Lemon beneficial effects: dyspepsia, constipation, respiratory infections, asthma, rheumatism, arthritis, lowers blood pressure, helps with weight-loss, anti-cancer, acne, eczema, burns.
- Use organic raw hone, yoghurt and lemons.
- Use regularly for better effects

Precautions:

- Lemon may cause photosensitivity when used on skin
- Do not use if you are allergic to any ingredient
- Contact your doctor with any questions or concerns

Disclaimer: This does not replace medical advice. Check With Your Doctor for symptoms or worsening of condition.

Eczema (Atopic Dermatitis)

Dermatitis (eczema) is a condition including a group of diseases characterized by red skin and itchiness, as a result of skin inflammation.

It includes many types of dermatitis: atopic dermatitis and irritant/allergic contact dermatitis.

Atopic dermatitis is a chronic disturbance, with periodical flares. It may involve small or large areas of the body, or even the entire body, and it is most common in children.

Symptoms and signs:

- itching, which may be quite distressing, especially during nighttime
- dry, thickened, scaly skin, even swollen and raw as result of scratching
- red-brownish spots and small, elevated knots on the affected areas

Seek medical advice when the condition is distressing and persistent, and when the lesions appear to be infected.

Risk factors:

- too dry skin
- various chemical substances, such as soaps, solvents, detergents, etc.
- stress
- smoking and air pollution
- diet containing eggs, peanuts, fish, etc.
- infections

Recipe 100 - Honey and Cinnamon

Difficulty: +; Time: 5 minutes;

Ingredients:

- 1 teaspoon honey
- 1 teaspoon cinnamon

Preparation: Mix honey with freshly ground cinnamon.

How to take it: Apply locally and cover it with a clean gauze. After 1-2 hours, remove the gauze and wash skin with warm water.

Tips:

- Cinnamon properties: contains vitamins (A, B complex, C), minerals (calcium, iron, manganese, phosphorous), essential oils (cinnamaldehyde, cinnamyl alcohol, cinnamyl acetate), flavonoids (alpha- and beta-carotens, lutein, zeaxanthin, cryptoxanthin, lycopene); anti-oxidant, anti-inflammatory, antimicrobial, antifungal, analgesic, anti-spastic, anti-parasites, haemostatic, peripheral vasodilator, lowers cholesterol, reduces stress and fatigue, promotes healing, anti-cancer.

- Cinnamon beneficial effects: infections (respiratory, gynecological: leucorrhea, vaginitis; digestive: gingivitis, mouth ulcers, enterocolitis, amoebiasis), dyspepsia, GERD, gastritis, peptic ulcer, asthenia, depression, Alzheimer, regulates menstruation, eczema, helps with weight-loss.
- Use organic raw honey and cinnamon.
- Use regularly for better effects

Precautions:

- Cinnamon: not to be used in pregnancy and in breast-feeding women.
- Do not use if you are allergic to any ingredient
- Contact your doctor with any questions or concerns

Disclaimer: This does not replace medical advice. Check With Your Doctor for symptoms or worsening of condition.

Recipe 101 - Honey and Cucumber

Difficulty: +; Time: 15 minutes;

Ingredients:

- 1 teaspoon honey
- 1 small size cucumber

Preparation: Mix honey with peeled and grated cucumber.

How to take it: Apply locally with a sterile gauze, for 2 hours, 2-3 times a day.

Tips:

- Cucumber properties: 95% water, vitamins (A, B complex, C, K), minerals (calcium, magnesium, potassium, iron, phosphorous, molybdenum, selenium, zinc), flavonoids (quercetin, apigenin, kaempherol, alpha- and beta-caroten, lutein, zeaxanthin), triterpenes (cucurbitacin A, B, C, D), lignans (lariciresinol, pinoresinol); stimulates blood circulation, anti-oxidant, anti-inflammatory, hydrating, diuretic, astringent, dissolves uric acid and urates.

- Cucumber beneficial effects: high blood pressure, gout, arthritis, kidney stones, constipation, helps with weight-loss, detoxification. Skin benefits in acne, dermatitis, sunburns.
- Use organic raw honey and cucumbers.
- Use regularly for better effects

Precautions:

- Cucumber contraindications: severe high blood pressure, ascitis, and other conditions with fluid retention.
- Do not use if you are allergic to any ingredient
- Contact your doctor with any questions or concerns

Disclaimer: This does not replace medical advice. Check With Your Doctor for symptoms or worsening of condition.

Recipe 102 - Honey, Aloe and Liquorice Powder

Difficulty: +; Time: 5 minutes;

Ingredients:

- 1 1/2 teaspoon honey
- 1 teaspoon aloe gel
- 1 1/2 teaspoon liquorice powder

Preparation: Mix honey with aloe gel and the liquorice powder.

How to take it: Apply mixture on the face or affected area. After 15 minutes, rinse it with warm water.

Tips:

- Liquorice properties: contains vitamins (B complex, E), minerals (calcium, magnesium, phosphorous, silicon, iron, zinc, selenium), flavonoids (beta-carotene, quercetin), phenol, glycyrrhizin, thymol, glabridin, phytoestrogens; anti-oxidant, anti-inflammatory, expectorant, growth inhibition of *Helicobacter pylori*, anti-tumor, anti-microbial (also anti-Mycobacterial, antiviral), boosts immunity, lowers cholesterol.

- Liquorice beneficial effects: mouth aphtous ulcers, dyspepsia, gastric and duodenal ulcer associated with *Helicobacter pylori*, liver protection, rheumatism, gout, polyarthritis rheumatoides, menopause, pre-menstrual syndrome, chronic fatigue syndrome, pulmonary infections, pulmonary tuberculosis, acne, shingles, helps in HIV infection, prevention and treatment of cardio-vascular diseases.
- Aloe properties: contains vitamins (A, B12, C), minerals (calcium, magnesium, copper, zinc, phosphorous, manganese, selenium, chromium), phytosterols, phenols (aloin, emodin), hormones (auxins, gibberellins), enzymes (aliiase, bradykinase, alkaline phosphatase, amylase), salicylic acid; anti-inflammatory, anti-microbial, lowers cholesterol, boosts immunity, anti-cancer, analgesic, helps with cough, laxative.
- Aloe beneficial effects: skin disorders (acne, psoriasis, eczema, burns, wounds), genital herpes, dental conditions, gum diseases, mouth ulcers, high blood pressure, sinusitis, respiratory infections, asthma, colitis, irritable bowel disease, gastro-duodenal ulcer, viral hepatitis, malabsorbtion, constipation, adjuvant in diabetes, weight-loss.
- Use organic raw honey, aloe and liquorice.
- Use once per day for better effects

Precautions:

- Liquorice should not be administered during pregnancy, while under digitalis or steroids treatment or in case of renal dysfunction with impaired salt excretion. During the cure, a low salt diet is recommended. May cause body fatigue, kidney disorders, irregular menstruation, may interact with diuretics. Prolonged use may cause the retention of fluid in the body, high blood pressure, low blood potassium levels (hypokalemia), and cataracts. Use in 4 to 6-week cure, followed by 2 to 3-week pause.
- Aloe may lead rarely to constipation. Caution is advocated in those with liver, gall bladder and kidney conditions. May cause abdominal pains. Avoid in severe, sudden abdominal pain (possible acute appendicitis, bowel occlusion etc.). Avoid in pregnancy, breast feeding women. Do not combine with steroids (corticosteroids), digoxin, other antiarrhytmics, diuretics. If you are on anticoagulants (blood thinners), ask your doctor before starting a cure!!!
- Do not use if you are allergic to any ingredient
- Contact your doctor with any questions or concerns

Disclaimer: This does not replace medical advice. Check With Your Doctor for symptoms or worsening of condition.

Psoriasis

Psoriasis is a common, long-lasting skin condition, in which itchy, red patches and scales occur on the skin.

It progresses in flares, and they may affect small or large areas of skin, or may cover the entire body.

There are many types of psoriasis: plaque psoriasis (the most frequent form), guttate psoriasis, nail psoriasis, pustular psoriasis, erythrodermic psoriasis, inverse psoriasis and psoriatic arthritis.

Symptoms and signs:

- red areas of skin, topped by silvery-white and thick scales: psoriasis plaque
- cracked and dry skin, which occasionally may bleed
- pain in the affected area (itching, soreness, burning, etc.)
- whitened or yellowed nails, and crumbled, pitted, ridged and thickened nails
- painful, stiff and swollen joints

Seek medical advice when noticing the above symptoms, if the symptoms are distressing and impair the daily life, or if there is persistent, severe symptomatology.

Risk factors:

- stress
- smoking and excessive alcohol drinking
- obesity
- relatives with psoriasis
- bacterial and viral infections

Recipe 103 - Honey and Dried/Fresh Beer Yeast

Difficulty: +; Time: 5 minutes;

Ingredients:

- 3 teaspoons honey
- 1 teaspoon beer yeast
- 1 l water

Preparation: Mix honey with yeast and water. Store in the fridge.

How to use it: Apply locally with a sterile gauze, for 2 hours, 2-3 times a day.

Tips:

- Beer yeast properties: contains vitamins (B complex), minerals (potassium, magnesium, selenium, zinc, copper, iron), beta-1,3 glucan, glutathione, mannan, trehalose; improves blood circulation, balances blood pressure and cholesterol, boost immunity, anti-aging, helps with calcium storage, prevents constipation, helps with weight-loss, tonic, enhances concentration, decreases fatigue.

- Beer yeast beneficial effects: cardio-vascular diseases, peripheral artheriopathy, metabolic regulation, psoriasis, acne, seborrhea, alopecia, stomatitis, infections, neuro-psychiatric disorders (Alzheimer, Parkinson, dementia), osteoporosis, andropause, and menopause.
- Use organic raw honey and beer yeast.
- Use for 10-30 days, pause for 1 week, then may repeat.

Precautions:

- Do not use if you are allergic to any ingredient
- Contact your doctor with any questions or concerns

Disclaimer: This does not replace medical advice. Check With Your Doctor for symptoms or worsening of condition.

Recipe 104 - Honey and Turmeric

Difficulty: +; Time: 2 - 3 minutes;

Ingredients:

- 1 tablespoon honey
- 1 teaspoon turmeric powder

Preparation: Mix honey with turmeric powder and make a paste.

How to take it: Apply mixture on affected area, once per day. After 15 minutes, rinse it with warm water.

Tips:

- Turmeric properties: vitamins (B complex, C, E, K), minerals (potassium, calcium, magnesium, copper, phosphorous, zinc, iron, selenium, manganese), curcuminoids (curcumin, demethoxycurcumin), volatile oils (turmerone, zingiberene, atlantone), resins, proteins, sugars; anti-inflammatory, mood improvement, blood thinning, lowers cholesterol, modulation of the immune response, painkiller, in Type 2 Diabetes reduces blood sugar and diminishes insulin resistance, anti-cancer.

- Turmeric beneficial effects: infections, Alzheimer's disease, depression, arthritis, inflammatory digestive tract diseases, cardio-vascular diseases, obesity, psoriasis, autoimmune diseases (lupus, rheumatoid arthritis, etc.).
- Use organic raw honey and turmeric.
- Use regularly for better effects

Precautions:

- Turmeric contraindications: pregnant women, during menstruation. Side-Effects: nausea and diarrhea, lowers blood pressure, higher bleeding risk (especially combined with anticoagulants). If you are on anticoagulants (blood thinners), ask your doctor before starting a cure!!!
- Do not use if you are allergic to any ingredient
- Contact your doctor with any questions or concerns

Disclaimer: This does not replace medical advice. Check With Your Doctor for symptoms or worsening of condition.

Skin Infections

Recipe 105 - Honey and Yoghurt for Genital Yeast Infection in Women

Difficulty: +; Time: 5 minutes;

Ingredients:
- 2 teaspoon honey
- 1 teaspoon yoghurt

Preparation: Mix honey with the yoghurt.

How to take it: Use it once or twice daily, topically around the vagina area.

Tips:
- Yoghurt properties: contains *Lactobacillus acidophilus*, vitamins (A, B complex, C, D), minerals (calcium, magnesium, potassium), proteins; probiotic, maintains a more acidic environment, lowers cholesterol, boosts immune system.
- Yoghurt beneficial effects: acne, vaginal infections, intestinal infections, flatulence, constipation, lactose intolerance, osteoporosis, hypertension.
- Use organic raw honey and yoghurt.
- Use regularly for better effects.

Precautions:

- Do not use if you are allergic to any ingredient
- Contact your doctor with any questions or concerns

Disclaimer: This does not replace medical advice. Check With Your Doctor for symptoms or worsening of condition.

Chapter 11

Arthritis

Arthritis is an inflammatory condition involving the joint(s). It includes osteoarthritis, rheumatoid arthritis, and other types of arthritis such as gout or arthritis caused by infections and other conditions.

Osteoarthritis is the most frequent type, in which the joint's cartilage is broken down. In rheumatoid arthritis, the lining of the joints is involved, with subsequent joint damage. Gout is characterized by the forming of uric acid crystals in the joints.

Symptoms and signs:

- pain in the afflicted joint(s)
- swelling and redness of the joint
- stiffness and lower range of motion in the joint

Risk factors:

- aging
- female gender (in rheumatoid arthritis); male gender (gout, other types of arthritis)
- relatives with arthritis
- obesity
- previous joint damage

Recipe 106 - Honey and Cinnamon

Difficulty: +; Time: 5 minutes;

Ingredients:

- 2 teaspoons honey
- 1 teaspoon cinnamon
- 250 ml water

Preparation: Mix honey with freshly ground cinnamon in one glass of hot water.

How to take it: 30 minutes before meals, in the morning and at dinner time.

Tips:

- Cinnamon properties: contains vitamins (A, B complex, C), minerals (calcium, iron, manganese, phosphorous), essential oils (cinnamaldehyde, cinnamyl alcohol, cinnamyl acetate), flavonoids (alpha- and beta-carotens, lutein, zeaxanthin, cryptoxanthin, lycopene); anti-oxidant, anti-inflammatory, antimicrobial, antifungal, analgesic, anti-spastic, anti-parasites, haemostatic, peripheral vasodilator, lowers cholesterol, reduces stress and fatigue, promotes healing, anti-cancer.

- Cinnamon beneficial effects: infections (respiratory, gynecological: leucorrhea, vaginitis; digestive: gingivitis, mouth ulcers, enterocolitis, amoebiasis), dyspepsia, GERD, gastritis, peptic ulcer, asthenia, depression, Alzheimer, regulates menstruation, eczema, helps with weight-loss.
- Use organic raw honey and cinnamon.
- Use regularly for better effects

Precautions:

- Cinnamon: not to be used in pregnancy and in breast-feeding women.
- Do not use if you are allergic to any ingredient
- Contact your doctor with any questions or concerns

Disclaimer: This does not replace medical advice. Check With Your Doctor for symptoms or worsening of condition.

Recipe 107 - Honey and Caraway

Difficulty: +; Time: 2-3 minutes;

Ingredients:

- 1 1/2 teaspoons honey
- 1 teaspoon caraway seeds (actual fruits)

Preparation: Mix honey with caraway fruits.

How to take it: In the morning and in the evening, 30 minutes before meals.

Tips:

- Caraway properties: vitamins (A, B complex, C, E), minerals (calcium, magnesium, zinc, iron, copper, manganese), flavonoids (lutein, beta-carotene, cryptoxanthin), volatile oils (carveol, fufurol, carvone, etc.); lowers cholesterol, anti-oxidant, anti-inflammatory, antiseptic, helps with cough, anti-flatulent, boosts immunity, stimulates and balances the female hormonal activity, triggers menstruation, diminishes pre-menstrual syndrome, stimulates lactate production, vermifuge.
- Caraway beneficial effects: high blood pressure, respiratory and other infections, arthritis,

rheumatism, gout, dyspepsia, irritable bowel syndrome, antihelmintic (intestinal worms), reduced milk secretion, pre-menstrual syndrome, dysmenorrhea (irregular and painful menstruation).
- Use organic raw honey and caraway.
- Use regularly for better effects

Precautions:

- Caraway seeds contraindications: high doses may affect kidneys and liver.
- Do not use if you are allergic to any ingredient
- Contact your doctor with any questions or concerns

Disclaimer: This does not replace medical advice. Check With Your Doctor for symptoms or worsening of condition.

Recipe 108 - Honey, Ginger, Garlic and Apple Cider Vinegar

Difficulty: ++; Time: 7 days;

Ingredients:

- 500 g honey
- ginger (4 cm length)
- 15 garlic cloves
- 300 ml apple cider vinegar

Preparation: Blend garlic cloves with ginger, honey and apple cider vinegar. Store the mixture in a sealed glass jar in the fridge. Stir every 2-3 days with a wooden spoon.

How to take it: 2 teaspoons dissolved in a glass of warm water, in the morning 30 minutes before meal.

Tips:

- Ginger properties: contains vitamins (B complex, C, E), minerals (calcium, magnesium, phosphorous, potassium, sodium, zinc, iron), gingerols, zingerone, shogaols (volatile oils), beta-carotene, capsaicin, caffeic acid, curcumin, salicylate;

anti-oxidant, anti-inflammatory, antibacterial, antifungal, analgesic, anti-nausea, lowers cholesterol, choleretic, anti-cancer.
- Ginger beneficial effects: respiratory infections, asthma, heart disease, GERD, stomach ulcer, diabetes prevention and therapy, weight loss.
- Garlic properties: contains vitamins (A, B complex, C, K), minerals (calcium, magnesium, iron, manganese, potassium, selenium, zinc, phosphorous), thiosulfinates (allicin, methyl allyl sulfinates), ajoenes, sulfides, sulfoxides (alliin, isoalliin, methiin, garlicins), flavonoids (beta-carotene, lutein, zeaxanthin); anti-bacterial, anti-viral, anti-fungal, anti-inflammatory, anti-oxidant, anti-platelet activity, decreases cholesterol, lowers blood sugar, lowers blood pressure.
- Garlic beneficial effects: heart diseases, high blood pressure, various cancers, respiratory infections, sinusitis, asthma, gastric and duodenal ulcers, especially associated with *Helicobacter pylori*, liver cirrhosis, osteoporosis, improves performance and reduces fatigue, detoxifies the body of heavy metals.
- Apple cider vinegar properties: contains vitamins (B complex, C, pantothenic acid), minerals (calcium, potassium, sodium, iron, phosphorus), acetic acid, malic acid, pectin, polyphenols (flavonols, flavanols, tannins, anthocyanins, dihydrochalcones, hydroxycinnamic acids); boosts immunity, anti-microbial, anti-inflammatory, anti-oxidant, lowers cholesterol, lowers blood sugar, acts as anti-acid.

- Apple cider vinegar beneficial effects: in infections (sinusitis, sore throat, asthma, other respiratory infections, urinary tract infections, etc), allergies, arthritis, gout, cardiovascular diseases, improves digestion, prevents constipation, helps with weight loss, in skin conditions (acne, eczema).
- Use organic raw honey, ginger, garlic, and apple cider vinegar.
- Use regularly for 1 month for better effects, then pause for 2 weeks. May be repeated.

Precautions:

- Ginger should be avoided in pregnancy and breastfeeding. It may cause blood thinning. If you are on anticoagulants (blood thinners), ask your doctor before starting a cure!!! Precaution is advised when using blood pressure medication.
- Garlic: may lower Saquinavir levels and may interact with some anticoagulants and diabetes medication. If you are on anticoagulants (blood thinners), ask your doctor before starting a cure!!! May cause flatulence and nausea. Locally applied may lead to irritation, urticaria, anaphylaxis.
- Do not use if you are allergic to any ingredient
- Contact your doctor with any questions or concerns

Disclaimer: This does not replace medical advice. Check With Your Doctor for symptoms or worsening of condition.

Recipe 109 - Honey and Corn Silk (infusion)

Difficulty: +; Time: 30 minutes;

Ingredients:

- 4 teaspoon honey
- 4 teaspoon dried corn silk
- 1 liter water

Preparation: Infuse dried corn silk with 1 liter boiling water for 2 minutes, then filter it and let it cool. Mix it with honey.

How to take it: 4 cups per day, preferably 30 minutes before meals.

Tips:

- Corn silk properties: contains vitamins (A, B complex, C, E), minerals (magnesium, iron, zinc, potassium, phosphorous), betaine, flavonoids (tannins), alantoine, volatile oils, ergosterine, proteins (zeine, with high content of leucine and glutamic acid), starch; antispastic, diuretic, haemostatic, improves liver function, anti-inflammatory, astringent; in high doses, decreases blood sugar.
- Corn silk beneficial effects: kidney stones, urinary tract infections, prostatitis, cardio-vascular

conditions, arthritis, rheumatism, high blood pressure, dysmenorrhea, menopause, edema, ascitis, helps with weight-loss.
- Use organic raw honey and corn silk.
- Use regularly for 3 weeks for better effects, every autumn.

Precautions:

Corn silk: avoid in pregnancy, precaution in diabetes, hypertension (interaction with Captopril, Enalapril, Furosemid), simultaneous administration of anti-inflammatory drugs which lower blood potassium; can reduce the efficacy of warfarin. Seek medical advice before starting the treatment.

- Do not use if you are allergic to any ingredient
- Contact your doctor with any questions or concerns

Disclaimer: This does not replace medical advice. Check With Your Doctor for symptoms or worsening of condition.

Recipe 110 - Honey, Green Walnuts and Ginger

Difficulty: ++; Time: 1 month;

Ingredients:

- 700 g honey
- 200 g green walnuts
- ginger (4 cm length)

Preparation: Mix honey with chopped green walnuts, put the mixture in a sealed jar, and store them in a sunny place for a month. Stir every 2-3 days with a wooden spoon. After 1 month store in a dark place.

How to take it: 1 tablespoon in the morning before breakfast.

Tips:

- Walnuts properties: vitamins (A, B complex, E), minerals (magnesium, zinc, manganese, molybdenum, copper, iron), flavonoids (beta-carotene, lutein, zeaxanthin), proteins (contain L-arginine, which is an essential amino acid); anti-oxidant, anti-inflammatory, lower cholesterol, increase insulin production, laxative.

- Walnuts beneficial effects: prevention of cardio-vascular diseases, lower blood pressure, prevent macular degeneration and cataract, asthma, rheumatoid arthritis, psoriasis, eczema, improve depression, prevent gallstones, constipation, Type 2 diabetes, great for hair and skin.
- Ginger properties: contains vitamins (B complex, C, E), minerals (calcium, magnesium, phosphorous, potassium, sodium, zinc, iron), gingerols, zingerone, shogaols (volatile oils), beta-carotene, capsaicin, caffeic acid, curcumin, salicylate; anti-oxidant, anti-inflammatory, antibacterial, antifungal, analgesic, anti-nausea, lowers cholesterol, choleretic, anti-cancer.
- Ginger beneficial effects: respiratory infections, asthma, heart disease, GERD, stomach ulcer, diabetes prevention and therapy, weight loss.
- Use organic raw honey and walnuts.

Precautions:

- Walnuts: may trigger allergy, even anaphylaxis; when used on skin may cause rash; may cause loose stools.
- Ginger should be avoided in pregnancy and breastfeeding. It may cause blood thinning. If you are on anticoagulants (blood thinners), ask your doctor before starting a cure!!! Precaution is advised when using blood pressure medication.
- Garlic: may lower Saquinavir levels and may interact with some anticoagulants and diabetes medication. If you are on anticoagulants (blood thinners), ask your doctor before starting a cure!!!

May cause flatulence and nausea. Locally applied may lead to irritation, urticaria, anaphylaxis.
- Do not use if you are allergic to any ingredient
- Contact your doctor with any questions or concerns

Disclaimer: This does not replace medical advice. Check With Your Doctor for symptoms or worsening of condition.

Recipe 111 - Honey and Liquorice (macerate)

Difficulty: ++; Time: 11 hours;

Ingredients:

- 3 teaspoons honey
- 3 teaspoons powder liquorice
- 500 ml water

Preparation: Macerate 3 teaspoons powdered liquorice in 250 ml water for 10 hours overnight, then filter it in the morning. Mix the filtered plant residue with 250 ml boiled water and let it cool. Mix the two solutions, add the honey and stir thoroughly. Store in the fridge.

How to take it: 1 cup twice a day, 30 minutes before meals, not longer than 1 month.

Tips:

- Liquorice properties: contains vitamins (B complex, E), minerals (calcium, magnesium, phosphorous, silicon, iron, zinc, selenium), flavonoids (beta-carotene, quercetin), phenol, glycyrrhizin, thymol, glabridin, phytoestrogens; anti-oxidant, anti-inflammatory, expectorant, growth inhibition of *Helicobacter pylori,* anti-tumor, anti-microbial

(also anti-Mycobacterial, antiviral), boosts immunity, lowers cholesterol.
- Liquorice beneficial effects: mouth aphtous ulcers, dyspepsia, gastric and duodenal ulcer associated with *Helicobacter pylori*, liver protection, rheumatism, gout, polyarthritis rheumatoides, menopause, pre-menstrual syndrome, chronic fatigue syndrome, pulmonary infections, pulmonary tuberculosis, acne, shingles, helps in HIV infection, prevention and treatment of cardio-vascular diseases.
- Use organic raw honey and liquorice.
- Use regularly for better effects

Precautions:

- Liquorice should not be administered during pregnancy, while under digitalis or steroids treatment or in case of renal dysfunction with impaired salt excretion. During the cure, a low salt diet is recommended. May cause body fatigue, kidney disorders, irregular menstruation, may interact with diuretics. Prolonged use may cause the retention of fluid in the body, high blood pressure, low blood potassium levels (hypokalemia), and cataracts.
- Do not use if you are allergic to any ingredient
- Contact your doctor with any questions or concerns

Disclaimer: This does not replace medical advice. Check With Your Doctor for symptoms or worsening of condition.

Chapter 12

Anemia

Anemia is a condition characterized by a reduced number of healthy red blood cells, able to carry oxygen. The result is diminished supply of oxygen for the body's tissues. There are many types of anemia, each with different underlying causes.

Symptoms and signs:

- weakness and fatigue
- dizziness, headache
- pale skin
- palpitations, chest pain
- shortness of breath

Seek medical advice if you experience fatigue or other anemia symptoms, because that could indicate a serious underlying disease.

Risk factors:

- diet low in iron, folate and vitamin B12
- alcoholism
- relatives with certain types of anemia
- intestinal conditions which cause malabsorption
- chronic diseases (kidney failure, cancer etc.)
- menstruation and other chronic blood loss (ulcer)

Recipe 112 - Honey, Aloe and Red Wine

Difficulty: ++; Time: 7 days;

Ingredients:

- 500 g honey
- 300 g aloe leaves (3-5 years old)
- 700 ml red wine

Preparation: Grind the aloe leaves and mix them with honey and red wine. Put the mixture in a sealed glass jar in the fridge. Let it macerate for 7 days.

How to take it: 1 tablespoon 3 times a day, 30 minutes before meals.

Tips:

- Aloe properties: contains vitamins (A, B12, C), minerals (calcium, magnesium, copper, zinc, phosphorous, manganese, selenium, chromium), phytosterols, phenols (aloin, emodin), hormones (auxins, gibberellins), enzymes (aliiase, bradykinase, alkaline phosphatase, amylase), salicylic acid; anti-inflammatory, anti-microbial, lowers cholesterol, boosts immunity, anti-cancer, analgesic, helps with cough, laxative.

- Aloe beneficial effects: skin disorders (acne, psoriasis, eczema, burns, wounds), genital herpes, dental conditions, gum diseases, mouth ulcers, high blood pressure, sinusitis, respiratory infections, asthma, colitis, irritable bowel disease, gastro-duodenal ulcer, viral hepatitis, malabsorbtion, constipation, adjuvant in diabetes, weight-loss.
- Use organic raw honey, aloe and red wine.
- Use regularly for better effects.

Precautions:

- Aloe may seldom lead to constipation. Caution is advocated in those with liver, gall bladder and kidney conditions. May cause abdominal pains. Avoid in severe, sudden abdominal pain (possible acute appendicitis, bowel occlusion etc.). Avoid in pregnancy, breast feeding women. Do not combine with steroids (corticosteroids), digoxin, other antiarrhytmics, diuretics. If you are on anticoagulants (blood thinners), ask your doctor before starting a cure!!!
- Do not use if you are allergic to any ingredient
- Contact your doctor with any questions or concerns

Disclaimer: This does not replace medical advice. Check With Your Doctor for symptoms or worsening of condition.

Recipe 113 - Honey and Milk

Difficulty: +; Time: 2 - 3 minutes;

Ingredients:

- 1 tablespoon honey
- 1 glass of milk

Preparation: Mix honey with lukewarm milk.

How to take it: 3 times a day, 30 minutes before meals.

Tips:

- Use organic raw honey and milk.
- Use in 20 to 40-day cures for better effects.

Precautions:

- Do not use if you are allergic to any ingredient
- Do not use if you have lactose intolerance
- Contact your doctor with any questions or concerns

Disclaimer: This does not replace medical advice. Check With Your Doctor for symptoms or worsening of condition.

Recipe 114 - Honey and Green Walnuts

Difficulty: ++; Time: 1 month;

Ingredients:

- 600 g honey
- 200 g green walnuts

Preparation: Mix honey with chopped green walnuts, put the mixture in a sealed jar, and store them in a sunny place for a month. Stir every 2-3 days with a wooden spoon. After 1 month store in a dark place.

How to take it: 1 tablespoon in the morning and at lunch, before meals.

Tips:

- Walnuts properties: vitamins (A, B complex, E), minerals (magnesium, zinc, manganese, molybdenum, copper, iron), flavonoids (beta-carotene, lutein, zeaxanthin), proteins (contain L-arginine, which is an essential amino acid); anti-oxidant, anti-inflammatory, lower cholesterol, increase insulin production, laxative.
- Walnuts beneficial effects: prevention of cardio-vascular diseases, lower blood pressure,

prevent macular degeneration and cataract, asthma, rheumatoid arthritis, psoriasis, eczema, improve depression, prevent gallstones, constipation, Type 2 diabetes, great for hair and skin.
- Use organic raw honey and green walnuts.

Precautions:

- Walnuts: may trigger allergy, even anaphylaxis; when used on skin may cause rash; may cause loose stools.
- Do not use if you are allergic to any ingredient
- Contact your doctor with any questions or concerns

Disclaimer: This does not replace medical advice. Check With Your Doctor for symptoms or worsening of condition.

Recipe 115 - Honey, Walnuts and Lemon

Difficulty: +; Time: 10 minutes;

Ingredients:
- 600 g honey
- 500 g walnuts
- juice from 2 lemons

Preparation: Mix honey with crushed walnuts and lemon juice, put the mixture in a sealed jar, and store it in the fridge.

How to take it: 1 teaspoon 3 times a day, 30 minutes before meals.

Tips:

• Walnuts properties: vitamins (A, B complex, E), minerals (magnesium, zinc, manganese, molybdenum, copper, iron), flavonoids (beta-carotene, lutein, zeaxanthin), proteins (contain L-arginine, which is an essential amino acid); anti-oxidant, anti-inflammatory, lower cholesterol, increase insulin production, laxative.

• Walnuts beneficial effects: prevention of cardio-vascular diseases, lower blood pressure, prevent macular degeneration and cataract,

asthma, rheumatoid arthritis, psoriasis, eczema, improve depression, prevent gallstones, constipation, Type 2 diabetes, great for hair and skin.
- Lemon properties: contains vitamins (A, B complex, C, E), minerals (calcium, magnesium, potassium, copper, manganese, zinc, iron), flavonoids (naringin, naringenin, hesperetin, alfa- and beta-carotenes, lutein, zeaxanthin, beta-cryptoxanthin, tannins), terpenes, citric acid, fibers; anti-oxidant, anti-inflammatory, anti-bacterial, antifungal, antiseptic, immune system booster.
- Lemon beneficial effects: dyspepsia, constipation, respiratory infections, asthma, rheumatism, arthritis, lowers blood pressure, helps with weight-loss, anti-cancer, acne, eczema, burns.
- Use organic raw honey, walnuts and lemon.
- Use for a month for better effects

Precautions:

- Walnuts: may trigger allergy, even anaphylaxis; when used on skin may cause rash; may cause loose stools.
- Lemon may cause photosensitivity when used on skin.
- Do not use if you are allergic to any ingredient
- Contact your doctor with any questions or concerns

Disclaimer: This does not replace medical advice. Check With Your Doctor for symptoms or worsening of condition.

Recipe 116 - Honey and Red Beets

Difficulty: +; Time: 10 minutes;

Ingredients:

- 600 g honey
- 400 ml red beat juice

Preparation: Mix honey with red beat juice. Store in the fridge.

How to take it: 1 tablespoon 30 minutes before meals, 3 times a day.

Tips:

- Red beets properties: contain vitamins (A, B complex, C, E, K), minerals (calcium, magnesium, copper, manganese), flavonoids (high content beta-caroten, lutein), high content in carbohydrates, betalains (vulgaxanthin, betanin); anti-oxidant, anti-inflammatory, detoxifying, lower cholesterol.
- Red beets beneficial effects: anemia, help prevent macular degeneration and cataracts, skin conditions, constipation.
- Use organic raw honey and red beets.
- Use regularly for better effects

Precautions:

- Red beets may rarely cause red or pink-colored urine (beeturia), especially in people with iron deficiency; less commonly color the stools in red. Avoid eating in excess - may induce kidney or gall-bladder stones.
- Do not use if you are allergic to any ingredient
- Contact your doctor with any questions or concerns

Disclaimer: This does not replace medical advice. Check With Your Doctor for symptoms or worsening of condition.

Chapter 13

Eye Diseases

Conjunctivitis (Pink Eye)

Conjunctivitis is an inflammation (infection) of the conjunctiva (the outermost layer of the eyeball and the inside lining of the eyelid). It is usually caused by an infection (viral and/or bacterial) or an allergy. The condition may affect one or both eyes.

Symptoms:

- Redness
- Pain
- Itchiness
- Burning sensation
- Conjunctivitis may combine with inflammation of the eyelids (blepharitis), resulting blepharoconjunctivitis

Risk factors:

- contact lenses used continuously over prolonged periods
- contact with infected persons with viral or bacterial conjunctivitis
- exposure to allergic agents (allergic conjunctivitis)

Recipe 117 - Honey and Water

Difficulty: +; Time: 2-3 minutes;

Ingredients:

- 1/2 teaspoon honey
- 1 teaspoon distilled or boiled and cooled water

Preparation: Dilute honey in water.

How to take it: Put 1-2 drops in each eye, 2-3 times daily. Continue as long as the infection persists.

Tips:

- Use organic raw honey (preferably Manuka honey)
- Prepare the mixture just before using.

Precautions:

- Do not use if you are allergic to any ingredient
- Contact your doctor with any questions or concerns

Disclaimer: This does not replace medical advice. Check With Your Doctor for symptoms or worsening of condition.

Visual Acuity

Visual acuity refers to the clarity or sharpness of vision. It is an estimate of visual performance, related to the discernment of spatial differences. It depends on neural and optical elements and processes.

Visual acuity is gauged by the ability to differentiate numbers or letters on a standardized Snellen eye chart.

Recipe 118 - Honey, Carrot and Lemon

Difficulty: ++; Time: 15 minutes, macerate for 2 weeks;

Ingredients:

- 500 g honey
- 500 g carrots
- 500 g lemons

Preparation: Blend carrots and lemons, then mix honey. Put in tightly sealed bottles in the fridge for 2 weeks.

How to take it: 1 tablespoon in the morning before breakfast.

Tips:

- Lemon properties: contains vitamins (A, B complex, C, E), minerals (calcium, magnesium, potassium, copper, manganese, zinc, iron), flavonoids (naringin, naringenin, hesperetin, alfa- and beta-carotenes, lutein, zeaxanthin, beta-cryptoxanthin, tannins), terpenes, citric acid, fibers; anti-oxidant, anti-inflammatory, anti-bacterial, antifungal, antiseptic, immune system booster.

- Lemon beneficial effects: dyspepsia, constipation, respiratory infections, asthma, rheumatism, arthritis, lowers blood pressure, helps with weight-loss, anti-cancer, acne, eczema, burns.
- Carrot properties: contains vitamins (A, B complex, C, E, K), minerals (copper, manganese, molybdenum), carotenoids (alfa- and beta-caroten, lutein), anthocyanindins, hydroxycinamic acid, high fiber content; anti-oxidant, anti-inflammatory, antibacterial, detoxifying, lowers cholesterol, lowers insulin resistance, boosts immunity.
- Carrot beneficial effects: prevents macular degeneration, improves vision, prevents heart disease, stroke, helps with gum and teeth disorders, improves digestion, anti-cancer.
- Use organic raw honey, lemon and carrots.
- Use once in spring and once in autumn for better effects

Precautions:

- Lemon may cause photosensitivity when used on skin
- Consumed in excess, carrots may color the skin orange (face, palms, feet). Avoid in small intestine inflammation, acute gastro-duodenal ulcer.
- Do not use if you are allergic to any ingredient
- Contact your doctor with any questions or concerns

Disclaimer: This does not replace medical advice. Check With Your Doctor for symptoms or worsening of condition.

Recipe 119 - Honey and Liquorice

Difficulty: +; Time: 2-3 minutes;

Ingredients:

- 1 1/2 teaspoon honey
- 1/2 teaspoon powder liquorice
- 1 glass warm milk
- 1/3 teaspoon butter

Preparation: Mix the ingredients together in milk.

How to take it: At bed time, not longer than 1 month.

Tips:

- Liquorice properties: contains vitamins (B complex, E), minerals (calcium, magnesium, phosphorous, silicon, iron, zinc, selenium), flavonoids (beta-carotene, quercetin), phenol, glycyrrhizin, thymol, glabridin, phytoestrogens; anti-oxidant, anti-inflammatory, expectorant, growth inhibition of *Helicobacter pylori*, anti-tumor, anti-microbial (also anti-Mycobacterial, antiviral), boosts immunity, lowers cholesterol.

- Liquorice beneficial effects: mouth aphtous ulcers, dyspepsia, gastric and duodenal ulcer associated with *Helicobacter pylori*, liver protection, rheumatism, gout, polyarthritis rheumatoides, menopause, pre-menstrual syndrome, chronic fatigue syndrome, pulmonary infections, pulmonary tuberculosis, acne, shingles, helps in HIV infection, prevention and treatment of cardio-vascular diseases.
- Use organic raw honey and liquorice.
- Use regularly for better effects

Precautions:

- Liquorice should not be administered during pregnancy, while under digitalis or steroids treatment or in case of renal dysfunction with impaired salt excretion. During the cure, a low salt diet is recommended. May cause body fatigue, kidney disorders, irregular menstruation, may interact with diuretics. Prolonged use may cause the retention of fluid in the body, high blood pressure, low blood potassium levels (hypokalemia), and cataracts. Use in 4 to 6-week cure, followed by 2 to 3-week pause.
- Do not use if you are allergic to any ingredient
- Contact your doctor with any questions or concerns

Disclaimer: This does not replace medical advice. Check With Your Doctor for symptoms or worsening of condition.

Recipe 120 - Honey, Walnuts and Lemons

Difficulty: ++; Time: 15 minutes;

Ingredients:

- 250 g honey
- 400 g walnuts
- juice from 4 lemons

Preparation: Mix honey with crushed walnut and lemon juice, and put them in a tightly sealed large jar. Store in the fridge.

How to take it: 1 tablespoon 30 minutes before every meal, 3 times a day.

Tips:

- Lemon properties: contains vitamins (A, B complex, C, E), minerals (calcium, magnesium, potassium, copper, manganese, zinc, iron), flavonoids (naringin, naringenin, hesperetin, alfa- and beta-carotenes, lutein, zeaxanthin, beta-cryptoxanthin, tannins), terpenes, citric acid, fibers; anti-oxidant, anti-inflammatory, anti-bacterial, antifungal, antiseptic, immune system booster.

- Lemon beneficial effects: dyspepsia, constipation, respiratory infections, asthma, rheumatism, arthritis, lowers blood pressure, helps with weight-loss, anti-cancer, acne, eczema, burns.
- Walnuts properties: vitamins (A, B complex, E), minerals (magnesium, zinc, manganese, molybdenum, copper, iron), flavonoids (beta-carotene, lutein, zeaxanthin), proteins (contain L-arginine, which is an essential amino acid); anti-oxidant, anti-inflammatory, lower cholesterol, increase insulin production, laxative.
- Walnuts beneficial effects: prevention of cardio-vascular diseases, lower blood pressure, prevent macular degeneration and cataract, asthma, rheumatoid arthritis, psoriasis, eczema, improve depression, prevent gallstones, constipation, Type 2 diabetes, great for hair and skin.
- Use organic raw honey, lemons and walnuts.
- Use for 1 month.

Precautions:

- Lemon may cause photosensitivity when used on skin
- Walnuts: may trigger allergy, even anaphylaxis; when used on skin may cause rash; may cause loose stools.
- Do not use if you are allergic to any ingredient
- Contact your doctor with any questions or concerns

Disclaimer: This does not replace medical advice. Check With Your Doctor for symptoms or worsening of condition.

Cataract

Cataract is a condition of the eye's lens in which it progressively becomes clouded. The result is poor vision and problems in recognizing faces and objects details, reading, driving, and night seeing.

Cataract occurs slowly in general, and can affect either one eye or both of them.

Symptoms and signs:

- diminished visual acuity
- clouded or glared vision and increased sensitivity to light
- double vision
- fading of colors
- impaired night vision

Seek medical advice if there are changes in your vision (flashes, double vision), especially sudden ones, as well as if there is sudden occurrence of eye pain.

Risk factors:

- lifestyle: smoking, alcohol abuse, obesity, exaggerated exposure to sunlight
- aging
- previous eye conditions (inflammation, injury) and eye surgery
- drugs: corticosteroids over long periods
- diseases: diabetes, hypertension, skin diseases (eczema, atopic dermatitis), hormonal disturbances (hyper/hypoparathyroidism, hypothyroidism).

Recipe 121 - Honey and Water

Difficulty: +; Time: 10 minutes;

Ingredients:

- 1 tablespoon honey
- 3 tablespoons distilled water

Preparation: Mix honey with water. Filter the mixture through gauze. Store it in the fridge.

How to take it: 3 drops in each eye in the morning and at bed time, for a year.

Tips:

- Use organic raw honey.

Precautions:

- Do not use if you are allergic to any ingredient
- Contact your doctor with any questions or concerns

Disclaimer: This does not replace medical advice. Check With Your Doctor for symptoms or worsening of condition.

Recipe 122 - Honey and Breckland Wild Thyme (Creeping Thyme) for early stages of Cataracts

Difficulty: +; Time: 10 minutes, maceration 2 months;

Ingredients:
- 400 g honey
- 100 g fresh creeping thyme

Preparation: Mix honey with crushed plants. Let the mixture to macerate for 2 months.

How to take it: 1 teaspoon, 3 times a day, 30 minutes before meals.

Tips:

- Creeping thyme properties: contains vitamins (A, C), flavonoids (tannins), saponins, volatile oils (thymol, terpinyl acetate, methylchavicol, carvacrol, borneol, caryophyllene, isobutyl acetate, α-pinene, 1,8-cineole, citral, citronellol, citronellal, p-cymene, linalool, geraniol, γ-terpinene, α-terpineol), serpiline; anti-inflammatory, anti-oxidant, antimicrobial, anti-helmintic, diuretic, choleretic, analgesic, mood improvement;

- Creeping thyme beneficial effects: respiratory and urinary infections, rheumatism, sciatic, depression, headaches, migraine, anemia, stimulates milk secretion in breastfeeding women, helps with weight-loss.
- Use organic raw honey and creeping thyme.

Precautions:

- Creeping thyme: contraindicated in pregnancy, angina, atrial fibrillation, inflammation of kidneys (pielonephritis), as well as in stomach and duodenal ulcers and liver inflammation (hepatitis)
- Do not use if you are allergic to any ingredient
- Contact your doctor with any questions or concerns

Disclaimer: This does not replace medical advice. Check With Your Doctor for symptoms or worsening of condition.

Chapter 14

Conclusion

We thank you for making it so far in reading this book.

As described in this entire work, honey is a valuable product, a true gold of nature, which humans have learned to use since thousands of years and they have done so unceasingly. The history section offers some insight, albeit not very extensive, into this temporal relationship.

And, even if, during the last few centuries, there was a decline in the general use of honey, particularly as a sweetener, during the closing decades, an increasing number of people became aware and interested once again in benefiting from it.

In order to facilitate this, we reviewed honey's characteristics, including the therapeutic features, properties which are more and more validated by scientific studies.

As you could notice, an impressive picture of honey's wonderful qualities resulted. In addition, we also portrayed the life and structure of bee colonies, so that now you may feel a bit closer to these fascinating and tireless insects, capable of such a complex and interdependent life.

Further, we presented a guide with numerous recipes for many diseases, which were also briefly and simply depicted. We never tired to warn about the importance of precisely following the recipes, as well as we kept advising that the treatment should be applied under medical supervision.

We hope you appreciated the information presented and already benefited from it or you will take advantage of it shortly.

In the end, we mention that the series continues with other bees' products, specifically pollen, propolis, wax, etc., as well as their use in therapy, cosmetics and household, including in the kitchen. So, don't miss the next volume!

Bibliography

Adel, Shirin P. R.; Prakash, Jamuna, Chemical composition and antioxidant properties of ginger root (Zingiber officinale), Journal of Medicinal Plants Research Vol. 4(24), pp. 2674-2679, 18 December, 2010. DOI: 10.5897/JMPR09.464

Adeleye, IA; Opiah, L., Antimicrobial activity of extracts of local cough mixtures on upper respiratory tract bacterial pathogens, West Indian Med J, vol. 52 (pg. 188-190), 2003.

Ali, AT; Chowdhury, MN; Al-Humayyd, MS, Inhibitory effect of natural honey on Helicobacter pylory. Trop Gastro-enterol 12:73–7, 1991.

Al-Himyari, F A, The use of honey as a natural preventive therapy of cognitive decline and dementia in the Middle East. Alzheimers Dement 5: 247. 2009.

Al-Jabri, Najwa Nasser; Hossain, Mohammad Amzad, Comparative chemical composition and antimicrobial activity study of essential oils from two imported lemon fruits samples against pathogenic bacteria, Beni-Suef University Journal of Basic and Applied Sciences Volume 3, Issue 4, Pages 247-253, 2014.

Al-Waili, NS., Effects of daily consumption of honey solution on hematological indices and blood levels of minerals and enzymes in normal individuals. J Med Food. 6:135–140, 2003.

Al-Waili, NS; Boni, NS, Natural honey lowers plasma prostaglandin concentrations in normal individuals. J Med Food 6:129-133, 2003.

Ames, BN; Shigenaga, MK; Hagen, TM, Oxidants, antioxidants, and the degenerative disease of aging. Proc Natl Acad Sci USA 90:7915-22,1993.

Azeredo, L da C; Azeredo, MAA; de Souza, SR; Dutra, VML, Protein contents and physicochemical properties in honey samples of Apis mellifera of different floral origins. Food Chem 80:249-54, 2003.

Ball, David W., The Chemical Composition of Honey, J. Chem. Educ., 84 (10), p 1643, 2007. DOI: 10.1021/ed084p1643

Baro, L; Fonolla, J; Pena, JL; Martinez, A; Lucena, A; Jimenez, J; Boza, JJ; Lopez-Huertas, E, n-3 Fatty acids plus oleic acid and vitamin supplemented milk consumption reduces total and LDL cholesterol, homocysteine and levels of endothelial adhesion molecules in healthy humans. Clin Nutr 22(2):175–82, 2003.

Bashkaran, Karuppannan; Zunaina, Embong; Bakiah, Shaharuddin; Sulaiman, Siti Amrah; Sirajudeen, KNS; Naik, Venkatesh, Anti-inflammatory and antioxidant effects of Tualang honey in alkali injury on the eyes of rabbits: Experimental animal study, BMC Complementary and Alter-native Medicine, 9 October 2011. DOI: 10.1186/1472-6882-11-90

BISWAS, B K, Effects of Honey on Feed Consumption and Body Weight of Sprague-Dawley and Obese Rats. Journal of the American Association for Laboratory Animal Science 48 (5): 613. 2009.

Bogdanov, S, Characterisation of antibacterial substances in honey, LWT-Food Sci Technol 17:74–6, 1984.

Bogdanov, S, Nature and origin of the antibacterial substances in honey, LWTFood Sci Technol 30:748-53, 1997.

Bogdanov, S, PhD; Jurendic, T; Sieber, R, PhD; Gallmann, P, PhD, Honey for Nutrition and Health: a Review, American Journal of the College of Nutri-tion, 27: 677-689, 2008.

Bogdanov, S, Nature and origin of the antibacterial substances in honey. Lebensm. -Wiss -Technol 30:748-753, 1997.

Borugă, O; Jianu, C; Mişcă, C; Goleţ, I; Gruia, AT; Horhat, FG, Thymus vulgaris essential oil: chemical composition and antimicrobial activity, J Med Life. 7(Spec Iss 3): 56–60, 2014.

Busswrolles, J; Gueux, E; Rock, E; Mazur, A; Rayssiguier, Y Substituting honey for refined carbohydrates protects rats from hypertriglyceridemic and prooxidative effects of fructose. The Journal of nutrition 132 (11): 3379-3382, 2002.

Chaieb, K; Hajlaoui, H; Zmantar, T; Kahla-Nakbi, AB; Rouabhia, M; Mahdouani, K; Bakhrouf, A, The chemical composition and biological activity of clove essential oil, Euagenia caryophyllata (Syzigium aromaticum L. Myrtaceae): a short review, Phytother Res. 21(6):501-6, 2007 Jun.

Chu, Wing-kwan; Cheung, Sabrina C. M.; Lau, Roxanna A. W.; Benzie, Iris F. F., Herbal Medicine: Biomolecular and Clinical Aspects. 2nd edition, Chapter 4 Bilberry (Vaccinium myrtillus L.)

Cooper, RA; Molan, PC; Harding, KG, The sensitivity to honey of Gram-positive cocci of clinical significance isolated from wounds, J Appl Microbiol, vol. 93 (pg. 857-863), 2002.

Cooper, RA; Molan, PC, The use of honey as an antiseptic in managing Pseudomonas infection, J Wound Care, vol. 8 (pg. 161-164), 1999.

Crane, E, The world history of beekeeping and honey hunting. Duckworth, London, UK, 1999.

Cushnie, T; Lamb, A, Antimicrobial activity of flavonoids. Int J Antimicrob Agents 20 26:343-356, 2005.

Dasaroju, Swetha; Gottumukkala, Krishna Mohan, Current Trends in the Research of Emblica officinalis (Amla): A Pharmacological Perspective, Int. J. Pharm. Sci. Rev. Res., 24(2), nº 25, 150-159, Jan – Feb 2014.

Dustmann, JH, Über die Katalaseaktivität in Bienenhonig aus der Tracht der Heidekrautgewächse (Ericacea). Z Lebensm Unters Forsch 145:292-295, 1971.

Efem, SE; Udoh, KT; Iwara, CI, The antimicrobial spectrum of honey and its clinical significance, Infection, vol. 20 (pg. 227-229), 1992.

Eteraf-Oskouei, Tahereh; Najafi, Moslem, Traditional and Modern Uses of Natural Honey in Human Diseases: A Re-view, Iran J Basic Med Sci.16(6): 731–742, 2013 Jun.

Ferreres, F; Garciaviguera, C; Tomaslorente, F; Tomasbarberan, FA, Hesperetin C a marker of the floral origin of citrus honey. J Sci Food Agric 61:121-3, 1993.

Gheldof, N; Wang, XH; Engeseth, NJ, Identification and quantification of antioxidant components of honeys from various floral sources. J Agric Food Chem 50:5870-7, 2002.

Irish, Julie; Carter, Dee A.; Shokohi, Tahereh; Blair, Shona E., Honey has an antifungal effect against Candida species, Med Mycol 44 (3): 289-291, 2006. https://doi.org/10.1080/13693780500417037

Jarić, Snežana; Mitrović, Miroslava; Pavlović, Pavle, Review of Ethnobotanical, Phytochemical, and Pharmacological Study of Thymus serpyllum L., Evidence-Based Complementary and Alternative Medicine, Volume 2015 (2015), Article ID 101978, 10 pages. http://dx.doi.org/10.1155/2015/101978

Jayaprakasha, GK; Jena, BS; Negi, PS; Sakariah, KK, Evaluation of antioxidant activities and antimutagenicity of turmeric oil: a byproduct from curcumin production, Z Naturforsch C.;57(9-10):828-35, 2002 Sep-Oct.

Johri, R. K., Cuminum cyminum and Carum carvi: An update, Pharmacogn Rev. 5(9): 63–72, Jan-Jun2011. doi: 10.4103/0973-7847.79101

Khalil, ML; Sulaiman, SA, The potential role of honey and its polyphenols in preventing heart disease: a review, African Journal of Traditional, Complementary and Alternative Medicines, Vol 7, No 4, 2010

Kramer, S N; Levey, An older pharmacopoeia. Journal of American Medical Association. 155 (1): 26, 1954.

Kilicoglu, B; Kismet, K; Koru, O; Tanyuksel, M; Oruc, MT; Sorkun, K; Akkus, MA, The scolicidal effects of honey. Adv Ther 23:1077-1083, 2006.

Kumar, Raj; Kumar, G. Phani; Chaurasia, O P; Singh, Shashi Bala, Phytochemical and Pharmacological Profile of Sea-buckthorn Oil: A Review, Research Journal of Medicinal Plants, 2011.

Larson-Meyer, DE; Willis, KS; Willis, LM; Austin, KJ; Hart, AM; Breton, AB; Alexander, BM, Effect of honey versus sucrose on appetite, appetite-regulating hormones, and postmeal thermogenesis, J Am Coll Nutr. 29(5):482-93, 2010 Oct.

Lee, Seung-Joo; Umano, Katumi; Shibamoto, Takayuki; Lee, Kwang-Geun, Identification of volatile components in basil (Ocimum basilicum L.) and thyme leaves (Thymus vulgaris L.) and their antioxidant properties, Food Chemis-try, Volume 91, Issue 1, Pages 131-137, June 2005.

MAAREC (Mid-Atlantic apiculture research and extension consortium), Honey Bee Biology: The Colony and Its Organization; http://agdev.anr.udel.edu/maarec/honey-bee-biology/the-colony-and-its-organization/

Mardomi, Reyhaneh, Determining the Chemical Compositions of Garlic Plant and its Existing Active Element, IOSR Journal of Applied Chemistry, Volume 10, Issue 1 Ver. I, PP 63-66, Jan. 2017 DOI: 10.9790/5736-1001016366

Martins, Natália; Petropoulos, Spyridon; Ferreira, Isabel C.F.R., Chemical composition and bioactive compounds of garlic (Allium sativum L.) as affected by pre- and post-harvest conditions: A review, Food Chemistry Volume 211, Pages 41-50, 15 November 2016.

Mayo Clinic http://www.mayoclinic.org

Mercan, N; Guvensen, A; Celik, A; Katircioglu, H, Antimicrobial activity and pollen composition of honey samples collected from different provinces in Turkey, Nat Prod Res. Mar;21(3):187-95, 2007.

Meghwal, M; Goswami, TK, Chemical Composition, Nutritional, Medicinal and Functional Properties of Black Pepper: A Review. 1:172., 2012 doi:10.4172/scientificreports.172

Mikaili, Peyman; Maadirad, Surush; Moloudizargari, Milad; Aghajanshakeri, Shahin; Sarahroodi, Shadi,

Therapeutic Uses and Pharmacological Properties of Garlic, Shallot, and Their Biologically Active Compounds, Iran J Basic Med Sci. 16(10): 1031–1048, Oct 2013.

Miraj, Sepideh, Phytochemical composition and in vitro pharmacological activity of rose hip (Rosa canina L.), Der Pharma Chemica, 8(13):117-122, 2016. http://derpharma-chemica.com/archive.html

Miraj, Sepideh, Chemical composition and pharmacological effects of Sambucus nigra, Der Pharma Chemica, 8(13):231-234, 2016.

Molan, PC, The antibacterial activity of honey. 1. The nature of the antibacterial activity. Bee World 73:5-28, 1992.

Molan, PC, The antibacterial activity of honey. 2. Variation in the potency of the antibacterial activity. Bee World 73:59-76, 1992.

Molan, PC. Honey as an antimicrobial agent, In: Mizrahi, A. and Lensky, Y. (eds.) Bee Products: Properties, Applications and Apitherapy. Plenum Press, New York, pp. 27-37, 1997.

Moritz, Robin F.A.; Fuchs, Stefan, Organization of honeybee colonies: characteristics and consequences of a superorganism concept. Apidologie, Springer Verlag, 29 (1-2), pp.7-21, 1998.

Muenstedt, K; Voss, B; Kulmer, U; Schneider, U; Hübner, U, Bee pollen and honey for the alleviation of hot flushes and other menopausal symptoms in breast cancer patients. Mol Clin Oncol, 2015. DOI: 10.3892/mco.2015.559

Murosaki, S; Muroyama, K; Yamamoto, Y; Liu, T; Yoshikai, Y, Nigerooligosacharides augments natural killer activity of hepatic mononuclear cells in mice. Int Immunopharmacol 2:151-159, 2002.

Nabavi, Seyed Fazel; Habtemariam, Solomon; Ahmed, Touqeer; Sureda, Antoni; Daglia, Maria; Sobarzo-Sánchez, Eduardo; Nabavi, Seyed Mohammad, Polyphenolic Composition of Crataegus monogyna Jacq.: From Chemistry to Medical Applications, Nutrients 7708-7728; 2015. doi:10.3390/nu7095361

Najafi, M; Shaseb, E; Ghaffary, S; Fakhrju, A; Eteraf-Oskouei, T, Effects of chronic oral administration of natural honey on ischemia/reperfusion-induced arrhythmias in isolated rat heart. Iran J Basic Med Sci. 14:75-81, 2011.

Nel, A. et al., A Review of the Eurasian Fossil species of the bee apis, PalaeontologyVolume 42, Issue 2 Version of Record online: 21 NOV 2003

Nel, A.; Martınez-Delclòs, X.; Arillo, A.; Peñalver, E., A Review of The Eurasian Fossil Species of The Bee Apis, Palaeontology, Volume 42, Issue 2, Version of Record online: 21 Nov 2003.

Nemoseck, TM; Carmody, EG; Furchner-Evanson, A; Gleason, M; Li, A; Potter, H; Rezende, LM; Lane, KJ; Kern, M., Honey promotes lower weight gain, adiposity, and triglycerides than sucrose in rats, Nutr Res. 31(1):55-60. 2011 Jan. doi: 10.1016/j.nutres.2010.11.002.

Nguyen, Nhat Minh; Gonda, Sándor; Vasas, Gábor, A Review on the Phytochemical Composition and Potential Medicinal Uses of Horseradish (Armoracia rusticana) Root, Journal Food Reviews International Volume 29, Issue 3, Pages 261-275, 2013.

Omotayo, O.; Erejuwa, Siti; Sulaiman, A. ; Ab Wahab, Mohd S., Honey: A Novel Antioxidant, Molecules 2012, 17(4), 4400-4423; doi:10.3390/molecules17044400

Orsolic, N; Knezevic, AH; Sver, L; Terzic, S; Heckenberger, BK; Basic, I, Influence of honey bee products on transplantable murine tumours. Vet Comp Oncology 1:216-226, 2003.

Orsolic, N; Basic, I, Honey as a cancer-preventive agent. Periodicum Biolog 106:397-401, 2004.

Pereira, José Alberto; Oliveira, Ivo; Sousa, Anabela; Ferreira, Isabel C.F.R.; Bento, Albino; Estevinho, Letícia, Bioactive properties and chemical composition of six walnut (Juglans regia L.) cultivars, Food and Chemical Toxicology, Volume 46, Issue 6, Pages 2103-2111, June 2008.

Postmes, T, The treatment of burns and other wounds with honey. In Munn P, Jones R (ed): "Honey and healing." Cardiff: IBRA International Bee Research Association, pp 41-47, 2001.

Rao, Pasupuleti Visweswara; Gan, Siew Hua; Cinnamon, A Multifaceted Medicinal Plant, Evidence-Based Complementary and Alternative Medicine, Volume 2014 http://dx.doi.org/10.1155/2014/642942

Roman, Ioana; Stănilă, Andreea; Stănilă, Sorin, Bioactive compounds and antioxidant activity of Rosa canina L. biotypes from spontaneous flora of Transylvania, Chem Cent J. 7: 73, Apr 23, 2013; doi: 10.1186/1752-153X-7-73.

Russell, KM; Molan, PC; Wilkins, AL; Holland, PT, Identification of some antibacterial constituents of New Zealand Manuka honey. J Agric Food Chem 18 38:10-13, 1988.

Sharma, Krishan Datt; Karki, Swati; Thakur, Narayan Singh; Attri, Surekha, Chemical composition, functional properties and processing of carrot - a review, J

Food Sci Technol. 49(1): 22–32, 2012 Feb. doi: 10.1007/s13197-011-0310-7

Shimazawa, M; Chikamatsu, S; Morimoto, N; Mishima, S; Nagai, H; Hara, H, Neuroprotection by Brazilian green propolis against in vitro and in vivo ischemic neuronal damage. eCAM. 2:201–7, 2005.

da Silva, PM; Gauche, C; Gonzaga, LV; Costa, AC; Fett, R, Honey: Chemical composition, stability and authenticity, Food Chem. Apr 1;196:309-23, 2016 doi: 10.1016/j.food-chem.2015.09.051.

Stanojević, Ljiljana P.; Stanković, Mihajlo Z.; Cvetković, Dragan J.; Danilović, Bojana R.; Stanojević, Jelena S., Dill (Anethum graveolens L.) seeds essential oil as a potential natural antioxidant and antimicrobial agent, BIOLOGICA NYSSANA 7 (1): 31-39, September 2016.

Surjushe, Amar; Vasani, Resham; Saple, D G, Aloe Vera: A Short Review, Indian J Dermatol. 53(4): 163–166, 2008. doi: 10.4103/0019-5154.44785

Swellam, T; Miyanaga, N; Onozawa, M; Hattori, K; Kawai, K; Shimazui, T; Akaza, H, Antineoplastic activity of honey in an experimental bladder cancer implantation model: in vivo and in vitro studies. Int J Urol 10:213-219, 2003.

Tanase, Nicolae, The Language of Honey, A Dictionary of Honey Varieties and Their Health Benefits, 2017.

The World's Healthiest Foods. whfoods.org

Theunissen, F; Grobler, S; Gedalia, I. The antifungal action of three South African honeys on Candida albicans, Apidologie, vol. 32 (pg. 371-379), 2001.

Uysal, Burcu; Sozmen, Fazli; Aktas, Ozgur; Oksal, Birsen S.; Kose, Elif Odabas, Essential oil composition and antibacterial activity of the grapefruit (Citrus Paradisi. L) peel essential oils obtained by solvent-free microwave extraction: comparison with hydrodistillation, International Journal of Food Science & Technology, Volume 46, Issue 7, Pages 1455–1461, July 2011.

Viuda-Martos, M. et al., Functional Properties of Honey, Propolis, and Royal Jelly, Vol. 73, Nr. 9, Journal of Food Sci-ence, 117-121, 2008

Weston, RJ; Mitchell, KR; Allen, KL, Antibacterial phenolic components of New Zealand manuka honey. Food Chem 64:295-301, 1999.

Yang, B; Liu, P, Composition and health effects of phenolic compounds in hawthorn (Crataegus spp.) of different origins, J Sci Food Agric. 92(8):1578-90. 2012 Jun. doi: 10.1002/jsfa.5671.

Zadeh, Jalal Bayati; Kor, Zahra Moradi; Goftar, Masoud Karimi, Licorice (Glycyrrhiza glabra Linn) As a Valuable Medicinal Plant, International journal of Advanced Biological and Biomedical Research, Volume 1, Issue 10: 1281-1288, 2013.

Zeina, B; Othman, O; Al-Assad, S, Effect of honey versus thyme on Rubella virus 6 survival in vitro. J Altern Complement Med 2:345-348, 1996.

Zeina, B; Zohra, BI; Al-Assad, S, The effects of honey on Leishmania parasites: an in vitro study. Trop Doct (Suppl 1):36-38, 1997.

HONEY – THE NATURE'S GOLD RECIPES FOR HEALTH

Authors' Bio

Both *Mona Illingworth* and *Daniel Andrews* underwent a medical doctor training. Nonetheless, they have managed to retain a strong and fulfilling relationship with the nature, connection which began in the country during early childhood.

In order to hand over their knowledge, as well as the humankind thousands-years old information about the nature, they created the *Bees' Products Series*. "*Honey - The Nature's Gold Recipes for Health*" represents the first volume.

The second volume is already in the making.

They hope this series will make a difference in people's life.

Please direct eventual suggestions at the publishing house's e-mail: scarletleafpublishinghouse@gmail.com.